THERAPEUTIC GARDENS

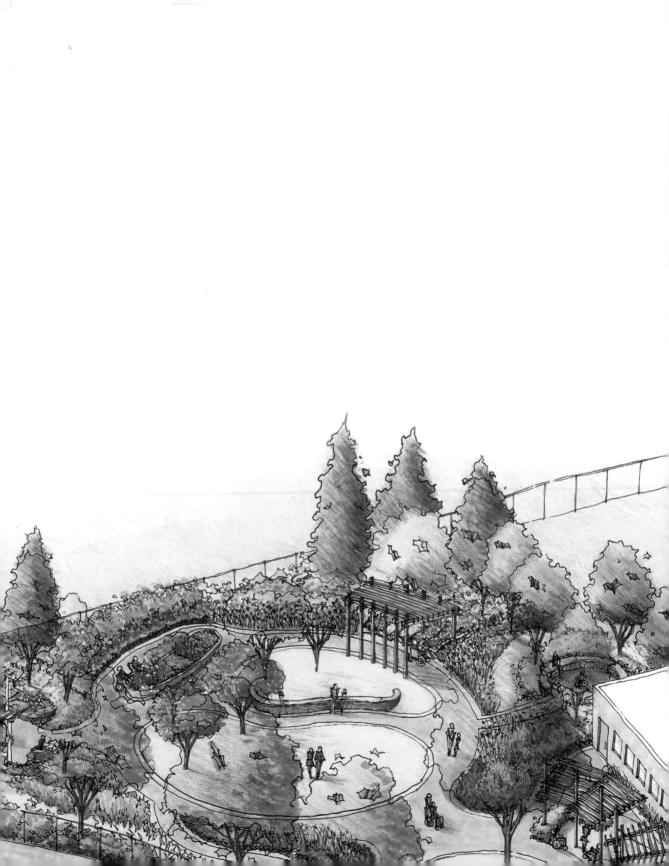

Therapeutic Gardens

Design for Healing Spaces

Daniel Winterbottom & Amy Wagenfeld

Timber Press
Portland ▪ London

Unless otherwise credited, all photographs are by the authors, and all drawings are by Daniel Winterbottom.

Published in 2015 by Timber Press, Inc.

The Haseltine Building
133 S.W. Second Avenue, Suite 450
Portland, Oregon 97204-3527
timberpress.com

6a Lonsdale Road
London NW6 6RD
timberpress.co.uk

Printed in China
Text design by Holly McGuire
Jacket design by Laken Wright

Library of Congress Cataloging-in-Publication Data
Winterbottom, Daniel M.
  Therapeutic gardens: design for healing spaces/Daniel Winterbottom and Amy Wagenfeld.—First edition.
     pages cm
  Includes bibliographical references and index.
  ISBN 978-1-60469-442-0
  1. Gardens—Design. 2. Gardening—Therapeutic use. I. Wagenfeld, Amy. II. Title.
  SB472.45.W56 2015
   712—dc23
                    2014024946

A catalog record for this book is also available from the British Library.

Contents

FOREWORD

Design is an expression of values. Through the designed environment—through the places we build to play, live, work, learn, and heal—we express our hopes and aspirations.

We are a product of nature. Over the course of thousands of years our evolutionary development, and eventually our cultural advancement, has been the result of endless interactions and adaptive responses to the natural environment. Our aspirations were intrinsically linked to a relationship with nature—where nature played the dominant role. In recent centuries that dynamic changed as technology and science gave us the opportunity to transform nature. Seen as a pendulum, our aspirations reflected an ever-increasing swing toward minimizing nature's influence in our lives. With our most recent technological advancements, the pendulum has swung so far that some question the need for nature in practically any form.

Others, however, including the authors and myself, happily understand that the pendulum is shifting back to the center, toward a more inclusive attitude to nature. Urban historian Sam Bass Warner calls it "rediscovering a common wisdom"; social ecologist Stephen Kellert eloquently says it is our birthright; biologist E. O. Wilson famously described it as biophilia, "the urge to affiliate with other forms of life." At its core is the fundamental link between humans and nature.

Probably nowhere is the need for a connection to nature more poignant than in times of illness and crisis, where balance and continuity is threatened and our sense of isolation and vulnerability heightened. A growing body of research is confirming that a connection with nature is essential to health and well-being. This benefit manifests itself in many ways, including reducing stress and depression, encouraging exercise and social connections, and accelerating healing with less medication. This book illustrates a concerted effort to balance our scientific and technological advancements with our intrinsic need for nature, in a way that is genuine, intimate, and immediate.

Such a shift in attitude and perspective demands a design response that is sensitive, adaptive, creative, and holistic. It requires us to reflect on the historical and cultural underpinnings of the art and science of healing as we embrace a future of dramatic and complex change—in climate, resources, and a multitude of other forces. It also requires that we practice design as a social art, with dialogue and in collaboration.

The designed environment can be instrumental in promoting health, both in helping individuals cope with ill health and in shaping individual choices that promote health. And this attitude about design can actually transcend any one particular scale: by putting individual human health on a continuum with environmental health, design can help coalesce individual choices into collective ones to make our communities, our cities, and our world more vibrant and equitable.

David Kamp, FASLA, LF, NA
Principal, Dirtworks, PC

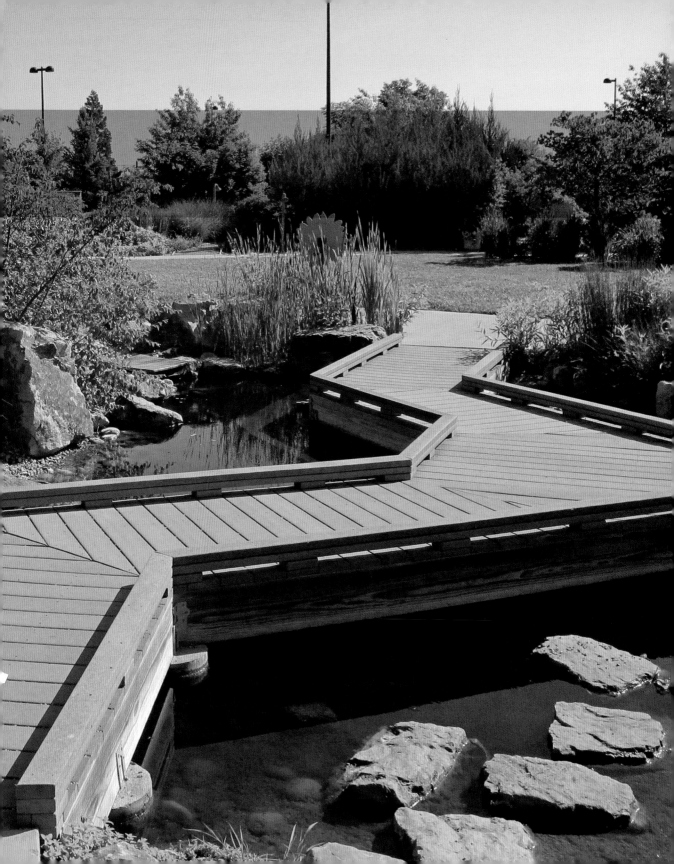

INTRODUCTION

Urban GreenWorks, a Miami-based nonprofit, develops productive green spaces for inner-city neighborhoods, connecting at-risk individuals to natural processes. The premise? By nurturing the landscape, clients are healing themselves.

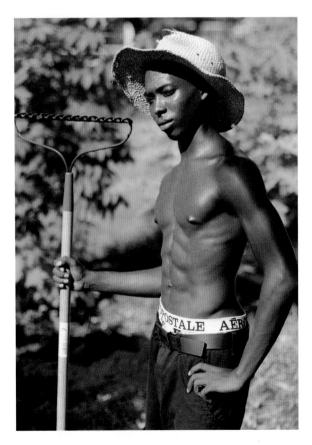

The routine of a typical weekday morning is interrupted, our attention caught by conversational voices on the radio. The intimate stories told by these anonymous people cause us to smile, to marvel, and sometimes to weep. Public radio employs the simple yet enduring medium of story-telling to illuminate and awaken. As they unfold in all their individuality, the stories we hear there—of resilience, acceptance, and devotion in the face of adversity—communicate the human struggle to overcome inequity, trauma, illness, or even fate; they draw generations together, to preserve the roots of a culture and nurture a sense of pride and belonging; they reveal a deeper understanding of human experience and document the power of place to shape our perspectives and life journeys. In listening, not just hearing, we bear witness to extraordinary displays of empathy, compassion, strength, courage, determination, and forgiveness. Each emotionally inspiring story illustrates the depth of humanity, rekindled by trying circumstances.

In the course of our work, we have discovered similar stories, stories shared while in the garden, by those with cancer, HIV/AIDS, physical challenges, or mental illness; by veterans, inmates, or the homeless; by the survivors of ethnic cleansing and torture; by the elderly facing the end of life. Each and every storyteller offers poignant examples of what nature means to him or her. It is what therapists hear and witness every day in the garden from those experiencing trauma, injury, and illness. Shared through intimate conversations, these stories provide motivation to design and evaluate therapeutic or healing gardens, to document further their benefits, and to educate people about them. The garden is sanctuary, a place to grieve and escape, to regain focus, hope, and strength, or to reconnect with family or one's former self. These gardens are not only relevant for those in hospitals, senior care facilities, or medical clinics; they also serve populations in need at schools, prisons, and community gardens.

Gardens can and do restore our state of health. They have the capacity to restore the body, mind, and spirit; and based on a growing body of evidence-based research, this can be said with conviction and proof. If being in a garden positively contributes to the healing and restorative process, who is it that needs a therapeutic garden and why? Many people who have experienced the benefits of gardens and nature will tell you that everyone needs a therapeutic garden. Others believe that people who are clinically unwell in body or mind are the only ones in need of a therapeutic garden. We believe that everyone needs easy access and proximity to nature and deserves this sacred connection that affords significant health benefits. Humans are hardwired to connect with the natural world. We have an evolutionary need to affiliate with nature. Originally, it was key to our survival; it is now part of our humanity.

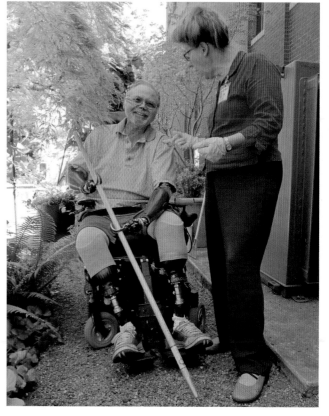

Gardening can reconnect the underserved and marginalized with their cultural roots and heritage, nurturing resilience and a sense of coherence.

While everyone needs and deserves safe, easy, and unencumbered access to healing nature, we return to a central question: is every garden a therapeutic garden? For now, consider this simple yet eloquent quote: "Gardens are where people and the land come together in the most inspiring way" (Rodale 1987). Some key words here—"people," "land," "come together," "inspiring"—will factor significantly in ongoing discussions about therapeutic gardens and the lives of those who are nourished by them. Being in nature has the capacity to bring people together, mediate social strife, renew one's energy and capacity, and nourish the senses. As humans, we find inspiration and consolation in nature; we grow stronger, learn, reflect, and refocus in the refuge it provides.

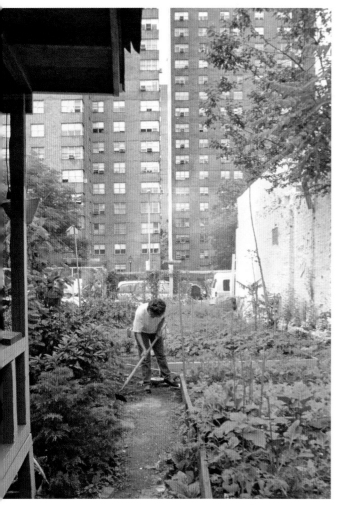

Engaging in physical activities in a garden, whether self-initiated or as part of a formal therapy program, is a highly motivating sensorial alternative to traditional routines.

For the Sake of Our Public Health

The multitude of public health issues we face are documented in our media daily. Childhood obesity rates may have stalled, but adult obesity and the diagnosis of autism is on the rise. Veterans are returning home from combat with shattering physical and emotional wounds, families are forgetting how to play together, children spend less and less time outside, food insecurity and hunger are affecting millions, and violent crime is entrenched in many neighborhoods and reducing the quality of life for their populaces. A common thread running through these seemingly disparate issues is lack of access to nature. Through universally accessible garden design that addresses the needs of diverse user groups, design teams have an unprecedented opportunity to play an active role in reducing the impacts of these public health issues. This book focuses on issues impacting the health of society and the role of therapeutic gardens in ameliorating some of their ill effects.

Sense of coherence, a concept developed by Aaron Antonovsky (1987, 1996), is the degree to which people feel they have control over their lives. A sense of control is one of our most profound personal needs, and it aligns well with a predisposition to connect with nature. How we comprehend, manage, and cope with stress (and also find meaning in what we do and experience) are components associated with sense of control. Unpredictability, loss of control, or a diminished sense of control may lead to or exacerbate depression, anxiety, fear, and sense of pain. Sense of coherence can be looked at through a wider lens when applied to garden design, especially when designing for emotional restoration. We experience salutogenic effects when there is balance between stress

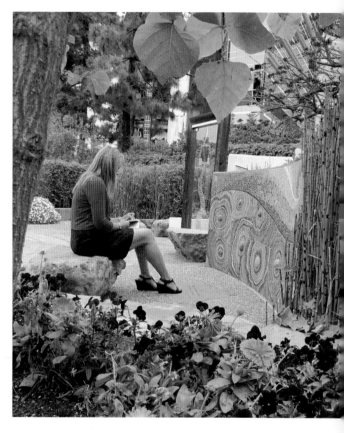

and coping, which balance in turn positively influences health. Salutogenic landscape design is intended to foster and maintain good health and resilience.

Connecting with nature in ways that are personally and culturally meaningful supports a sense of control. Being in well-planned, appealing outdoor environments has positive implications for health. Several research studies have found blood pressure and heart rate are lowered when exercising or socializing outdoors. Other research shows that exercising outdoors makes us feel better; for instance, those who run in green parks feel calmer and are more focused than those who run in urban settings (Bodin and Hartig 2003). Immersive walks (*shinrin-yoku*, "forest bathing") in a wooded area lead to lower cortisol levels, lower blood pressure, and increased sense of self-centering as compared to walks in an urban area (Park et al. 2010). Just like indoor exercising, outdoor exercising increases endorphin production (resulting in feelings of pleasure and happiness), strengthens muscles, and improves balance, but the outdoor environment is more motivating to many (Coon et al. 2011). Gardening burns up to 500 calories an hour, and doing heavy garden tasks like digging and hauling improves bone density (Turner et al. 2002).

Mental health benefits are also associated with nature-based therapeutic activities (Gonzalez et al. 2010). Gardening reduces stress, anxiety, and blood pressure (van den Berg and Custers 2011). Depressive symptoms and agitation are lowered. People feel calm when their internal heart rhythms synchronize with patterns of sound in nature, and they find the fractal geometries of branching patterns intrinsically satisfying (Sternberg 2009). Being in nature improves attention and sense of self-satisfaction; it diminishes aggressive behavior, increases empathy levels, and improves positive social interaction with others (Weinstein et al. 2009). Exercising for a minimum of 20 minutes a week, including gardening, is associated with better mental health and reduced risk of cognitive decline. Residents at skilled nursing facilities who spent an hour a day in the garden were more focused and calmer than those who spent that same hour inside,

Whether healing from physical or emotional trauma, meditative exercises can be an instrumental part of treatment, as in this 12-step garden.

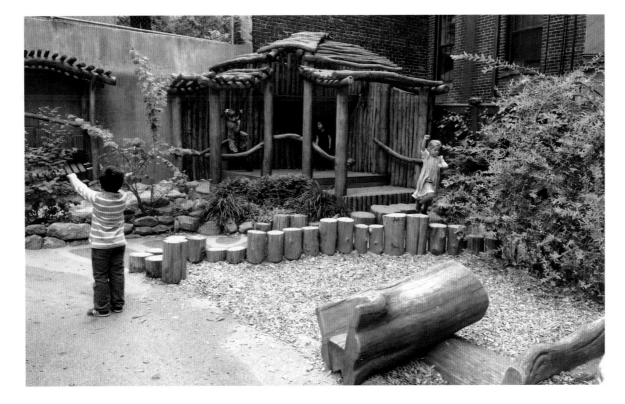

For children, outdoor play supports all aspects of development and engenders creativity and spontaneity.

resting (Ottosson and Grahn 2005). Those newly diagnosed with breast cancer show improved concentration and attentional capacity following two hours of interaction with a natural outdoor environment per week (Cimprich and Ronis 2003). We feel more positive and have a better outlook on life after spending time outdoors in nature. For many there also is a spiritual connection, one that calms, offering a centering and meditative quality to the experience of being in gardens.

A green outdoor space encourages more creative and active play and improves adult-child interactions, all qualities that are highly beneficial to healthy child development. Children with attention deficit hyperactivity disorder demonstrate fewer symptoms when they simply go outside and play for 20 minutes a day (Kuo and Faber Taylor 2004). Children who live close to nature experience a heightened sense of resilience; comparatively, they feel they are more capable and able to master challenges than their peers who do not have this same proximity to nature (Wells and Evans 2003).

Aggression levels are significantly diminished when nature is present outside apartment complexes in marginalized neighborhoods as compared to when there is none. There are fewer reports of crime, fear, incivility, and violence when people live in or near greener spaces. Gardens and gardening together can mediate conflict and increase conciliation. Compared to those living in or near barren spaces, people who live in greener areas are more social, know their neighbors, and experience a greater sense of belonging and less fear. People who live in or close to green spaces actually tend to live longer than those who do not (Mitchell and Popham 2008).

Some powerful positive secondary effects are also associated with access to nature. For instance, studies have shown that people recovering from surgery in rooms with brighter sunlight needed 22 percent less pain medication than patients in darker recovery rooms (Walch et al. 2005), and patients undergoing bronchoscopies had less anxiety when viewing pictures of nature at their bedside and listening to nature sounds before, during, and after their procedure (Diette et al. 2003).

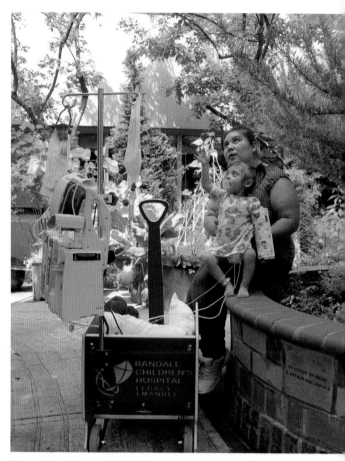

Being outdoors in a supported garden environment increases the sense of connection, escape, and hope.

What You Will Find in the Book

This book contains stories, guidelines, images, and drawings to use as inspiration and to support the design of therapeutic garden projects. We also include drawings of elements that are well suited for therapeutic gardens. Many of these elements are designed with physical and psychological rehabilitation in mind. Establishing collaborations between occupational therapists and designers at the onset of project design can better meet the specific user needs for the garden project.

Many books on therapeutic gardens focus on examples that are located in hospitals, long-term care facilities, and clinics. This book focuses instead on how a garden can be designed and used to achieve therapeutic outcomes for specific populations such as refugees, the homeless, and those with physical, developmental, and mental illnesses. It also focuses on specific types of gardens for learning, movement, sensory nourishment, reconciliation, and memorialization. This book complements the existing body of case study and research evidence and expands upon what is known by explaining how gardens are designed to support improved health and participation. Written by a landscape architect and occupational therapist, this book offers an interdisciplinary approach for the creation of therapeutic gardens where the combined strengths of both professions balance and support each other.

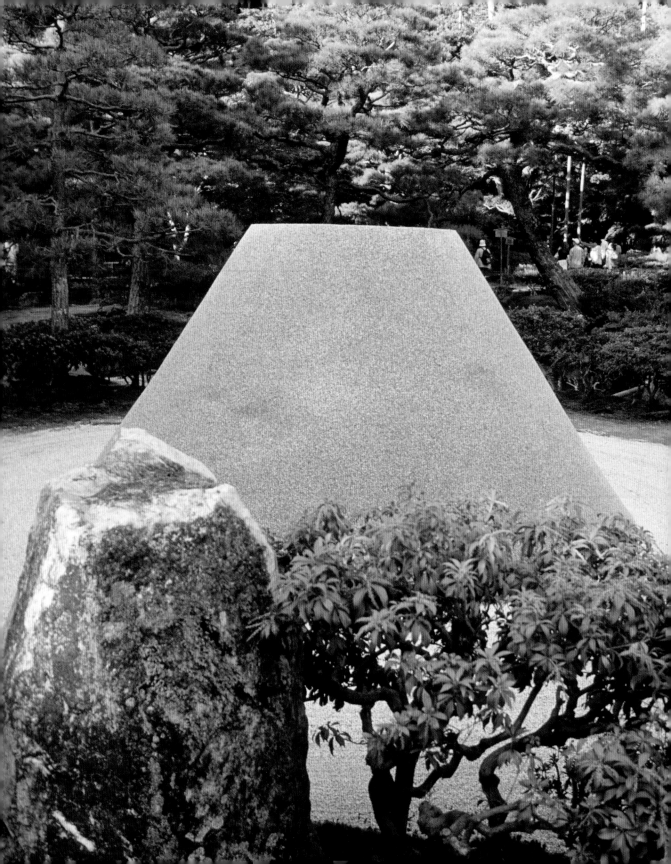

CHAPTER ONE
FOUNDATIONS

The framework of ideas underlying therapeutic gardens is best understood from three points of view. First is a look back through history at some gardens described either as healing or as centers for healing activities; the connection between nature and spirituality as associated with well-being is by no means a new concept. These examples across time and cultures also show how concepts of gardens, of nature, and of healing are mutable. The walled symmetry of many historic Western gardens reveals a longing for order and safety—protection from the threats of a wild, untamed nature. Today, by contrast, many living in densely built places try to reconnect to nature through gardens, turning their backyards, as nearly as possible, into "natural" habitats for wildlife. Ideas about health and treatment have evolved, too, along with the hospital environment and countless technological and medical advances.

Second is a look at theory and the growing body of scientific research on nature, people, and healing. Driven and tested by environmental psychologists, sociologists, healthcare providers, and architects striving to improve healthcare by designing more supportive facilities, these evidence-based studies reveal many general characteristics of space planning and nature interactions that can be applied to therapeutic garden design.

Third are the hands-on applications of those who work in the field, immersed in communities of need, to create therapeutic gardens. These are highly collaborative teams of landscape architects and designers, environmental psychologists, and therapeutic practitioners who know and respect each other's distinct approaches, language, and terminology. This maximizes the opportunity for both skillful design and nimble responsiveness to the varied and complex health challenges of users. The success of working together across disciplines is tied to an equality of interaction throughout the project, from conceptualization through design development.

When Hanley Denning brought her young students for their first visit to a park, she was struck by their transformation, by their expressions of joy and wonder as they chased insects and rolled in the grass. They were the children of the families working in and living near the Guatemala City garbage dump, and she, a teacher and social worker, had built a program, Safe Passage, to support their enrollment and success in school. She knew well that their situations of poverty, neglect, and abuse did not feature access to such beautiful natural places. Her new school was being developed on four acres of decommissioned garbage dump land. Hanley found a community partner in the University of Washington's landscape architecture design/ build program; they shared Hanley's belief that nature is healing and determined that her school would be surrounded by a green park and playscape, so that the children would learn and be nurtured by nature every day. Central to realizing Hanley's vision was to imbue every aspect of the design with nature and to dig deeply to understand the needs of the children and their families, so that the garden would help them learn and grow together in a safe and healthy way. Designed and built for communities under stress, these kinds of gardens are often known as therapeutic or healing gardens.

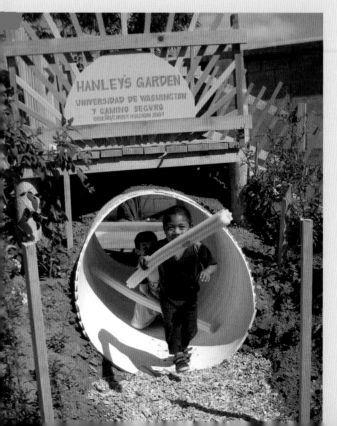

In "Hanley's Garden," children are free to invent and direct their play.

History

The temple at Epidaurus, on a hill with views to a pastoral landscape, fresh air, and natural springs, was a restorative center for healing in classical times, the best known of some two hundred temples to Asclepius, the Greek god of healing. The sick made the pilgrimage to its sanatoria for dream therapy, diet and exercise regimens, and baths. For the Greeks, the entire site was sacred. Structures were built in harmony with the landscape; the paths leading to it recognized and celebrated the natural features of hills, valleys, and views.

Persian gardens were cool and shady oases in the deserts of Iran, a manifestation of paradise or *pairi-daeza* ("beautiful garden enclosed by walls"). From grand to modest, paradise gardens were an essential feature of the Persian built environment, of public parks, and private homes and palaces. They were spiritually connected to a Zoroastrian

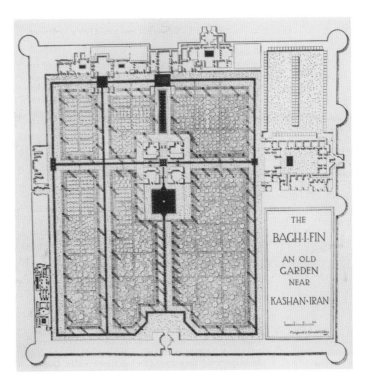

The simple geometric design of "an old garden near Kashan Iran."

belief in the four natural elements: earth (to grow plants), air (or heavens), water, and fire. The gardens were aesthetically connected to literature and poetry, carpet and textile design, miniature painting, music, and architectural ornamentation. All celebrated a reverence for trees and aromatic flowering plants, and water. The principle of their layout, the *chahar bagh* or foursquare garden pattern, has persisted for two millennia with widespread influence both to the East (e.g., the Taj Mahal in India) and to the West (e.g., the Generalife in Granada, Spain). The primary chahar bagh layout was a walled square with two intersecting water channels running north-south and east-west, dividing the garden into four parts.

Completed in 1590, the Bagh-e Fin, a UNESCO site, is the oldest existing garden in Iran, and it is an iconic iteration of the chahar bagh. Typically the gardens were inward-looking to inspire relaxation and reflection, eliciting

LEFT The cooling and sensorial qualities of Bagh-e Fin animate the garden while providing a calming, peaceful quality.

RIGHT A spiritual connection is innately evident at Kyoto's Saiho-ji, where time seems to slow, if not stop, at this mossy bridge over reflective water.

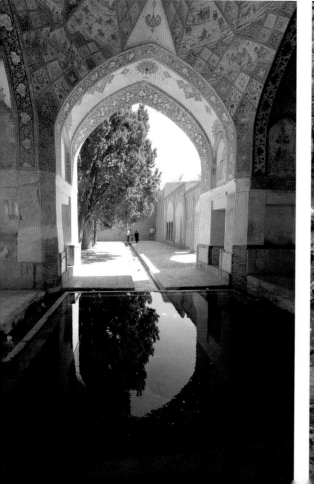

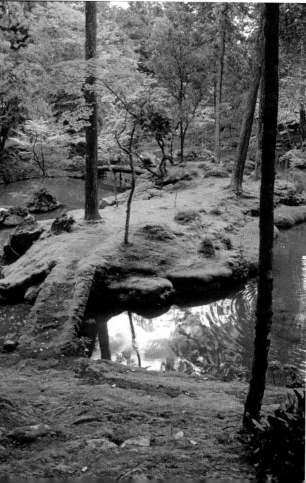

a response to nature through their sensual beauty. In the garden, nature was controlled, both in the geometric patterns of its layout and in the creation of its own microclimate. Sunlight reflected on water and shimmered on walls. The touch of cooling air was lofted by splashing sprays of water. Borders were thickly planted visual delights, and shelters accentuated the qualities of light, sound, and scent.

In Japan, gardens embody the ancient Shinto reverence for natural things; each *niwa* ("garden") is a piece of ground consecrated for worship of the spirits in every stone, tree, and spring of water. Saiho-ji is a garden in Kyoto, one of the earliest existing gardens influenced by Zen philosophy. Designed in 1339 and composed for contemplation, it is said to have been a response to the chaotic conditions of the time. Beauty is found in the irregularity and informality of unfolding natural processes, with an accent on the inherent forms, colors, and textures of stone, bark, leaf, and water. The large pond with crenulated shores and islands is surrounded by a laid stone strolling path, flanked by an undulating blanket of moss. Views through pines to distant views and landmarks give spatial depth and continuity to the journey and encourage a slow pace. The ever-changing prospects open the mind to calming reflection.

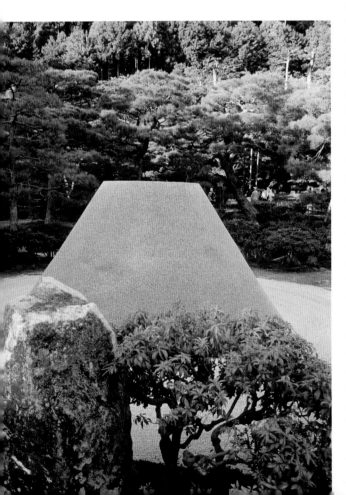

In stark contrast to the aesthetic of the verdant Saiho-ji, the dry garden at Ginkaku-ji, another Zen temple in Kyoto, inspires intensely focused meditation.

Cultures throughout history have treated illness with medicines derived from plants. Remedies have been etched into Sumerian tablets, written in hieroglyph on Egyptian papyruses, inked in ancient Chinese manuscripts, and illuminated in early medieval books. Much is revealed about medieval gardens and healing in firsthand accounts from European monastic communities, which held a large network of land holdings. Around 800, Charlemagne issued a plan for estate and monastery gardens throughout the Frankish empire, listing 89 plants, and in his *Hortulus* one Walifrid Strabo (808–849) describes a layout of raised beds with a trellis of climbing gourds and squash over a portico, complete with details of companion planting such as fragrant silvery-leafed artemisia, rue, and horehound, underplanted to protect the vines. The healing uses of each plant, for such

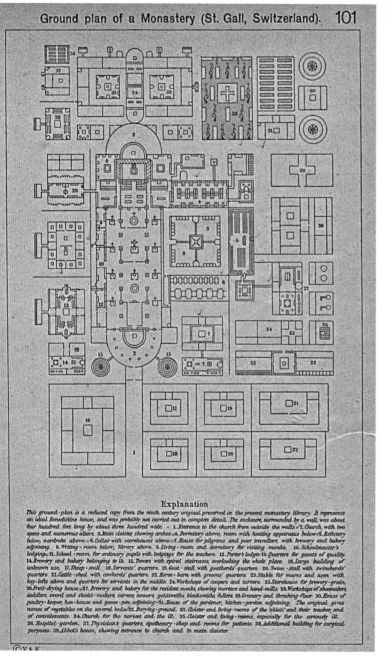

Ground plan of St. Gall.

conditions as hoarseness, stomach upset, gout, inflammation, chest pain, and poisoning, are carefully noted as well. Within the boundaries of monasteries, especially, a great variety of food, herbs, and medicinal plants was grown to sustain the community and its visitors. A typical garden layout of the ninth century is seen in the three gardens shown in the plan at St. Gall. The orchard garden, serving also as the monks' cemetery, held fruit and nut trees, including chestnut, hazel, quince, fig, apple, pear, plum, and almond. The kitchen garden featured 18 beds of garlic, dill, shallot, onion, leek, chervil, celery, chard, cabbage, poppy, parsnip, parsley, summer savory, and more. The herbularis, located next to the monk's infirmary in the upper left corner of the plan, was filled with what were thought to be medicinal plants—cumin, fennel, lily, lovage, mint, pennyroyal, rose, rue, sage, and black-eyed pea.

The work of maintaining the gardens was viewed as an act of devotion, tying the religious community together and meeting both physical and spiritual needs. A monastery's enclosed cloister gardens gave protection from the elements for meditative and prayerful walking. Open, simple greenery was a backdrop for a central sculpture or fountain, their own Garden of Paradise, with the fountain of water at its center representing the source of spiritual healing and eternal life. For many travelers to holy sites in the Middle Ages, care and sanctuary was given by church hospices along the numerous routes. In the healing of the sick, body and soul were treated as one.

The oldest known extant garden for medicinal plants is at the University of Padua, in Italy. It was founded in 1545 by the Venetian Republic to teach students how to recognize and use the plants, whose identification was not always certain (sometimes with deadly consequences). Some 1,800 species were grown, including many exotics collected worldwide—an advantage of proximity to Venice, a center of shipping trade. The five-acre garden was enclosed by a circular wall to protect against theft. Cleric Daniele Barbaro's original elegant design lays out a square within a circle, the square divided into quarters by two intersecting paths oriented to the cardinal compass points. Each of the four raised square beds featured a distinct (and distinctly geometric) planting scheme. A central pool and fountain, sundials, and other features were added over the years. By the 19th century, this walled garden had contributed much to the scientific disciplines of botany, medicine, ecology, and pharmacology.

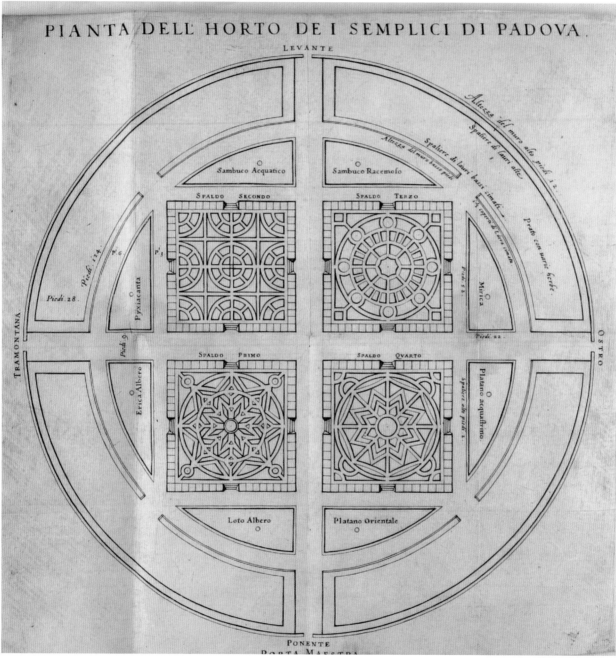

PIANTA DELL' HORTO DE I SEMPLICI DI PADOVA.

OPPOSITE The contained symmetry of the botanical garden in Padua was inward-focused, providing a meditative escape from the surroundings.

TOP An overview of the walled garden, here seen with the later addition of a central pool and fountain.

BOTTOM Worcester State Hospital looks out over a rural, almost pastoral scene of modest cottages and rolling landscape.

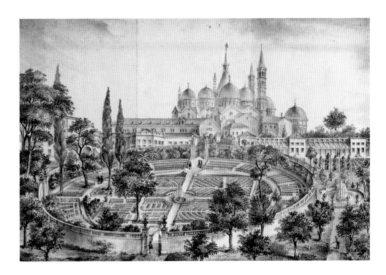

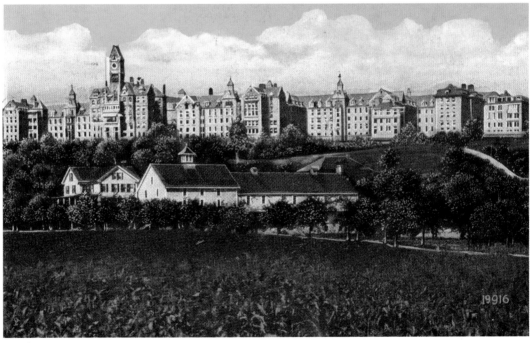

Now a UNESCO world heritage site, it still serves an important educational function within and beyond the university.

Also by the 19th century, in Britain and America, new ideas concerning the housing and treatment of the mentally ill were stirring. The movement was based on Quaker moral principles and belief in the nurturing powers of nature. Benjamin Rush, a physician at Philadelphia's Friends Hospital, was among the first to develop a program that used plants as a therapeutic modality. In Massachusetts, what is now the Worcester State Hospital was built according to psychiatrist and Quaker Thomas Kirkbride's 1854 plan. Its location was rural, offering sweeping vistas on a campus-like setting, and the extensive grounds included farmland tended by patients as daily exercise and productive work toward recovery of their mental health. A summary of the asylum farm account for 1893 lists the harvest, including 2,138 quarts of currants, 483 dozen eggs, and 496 quarts of milk. Similar accounts in Great Britain from Victorian asylums describe the opportunities of farm work as not only useful but socially engaging and stimulating experiences. As a Scottish commissioner reported, "For one patient who will be stirred to rational reflection or conversation by such a thing as a picture, twenty of the ordinary inmates of asylums will be so stirred in connection with the prospects of the crops, . . . the lifting of the potatoes [or] the growth of the trees" (Tuke and Savage 1881). Unfortunately, despite this shift in thinking, people with mental disorders were still poorly understood. Many ill-conceived treatment regimens involving harsh restraints and punishments prevailed. Nature as a cure was still the exception rather than the rule.

By the turn of the century, new ideas about humane, moral, and antiseptic treatment of the poor and infirm brought openness, fresh air, and sunlight to hospital designs. The Hospital de la Santa Creu i Sant Pau in Barcelona, Spain, incorporated these advancements with style. Begun in 1901, it was conceived as an arrangement of colorful pavilions in a quadrangular park with wide walkways, abundant gardens, and courtyards. Architect Domènech i Montaner believed beauty provided therapeutic value to help patients recover from illness. The finest artisans were hired, ornamenting the floors, façades, columns, and capitals in the floral modernist, or art nouveau style. A mosaic mural tells the history of hospital care. The landscaping served as a green matrix connecting what the architect described as a therapeutic campus, but unfortunately the original purpose of the gardens to enhance patient life was diminished over time

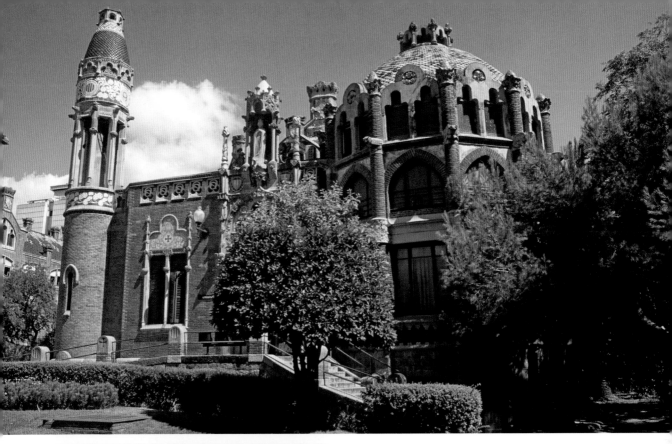

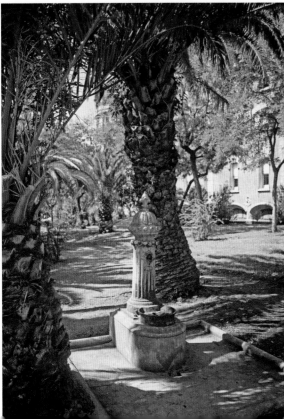

TOP Barcelona's Hospital de la Santa Creu i Sant Pau was the ultimate expression of aesthetic beauty inspired by nature.

BOTTOM This small remnant of the initial vision was appreciated by staff and patients until the hospital closed in 2009.

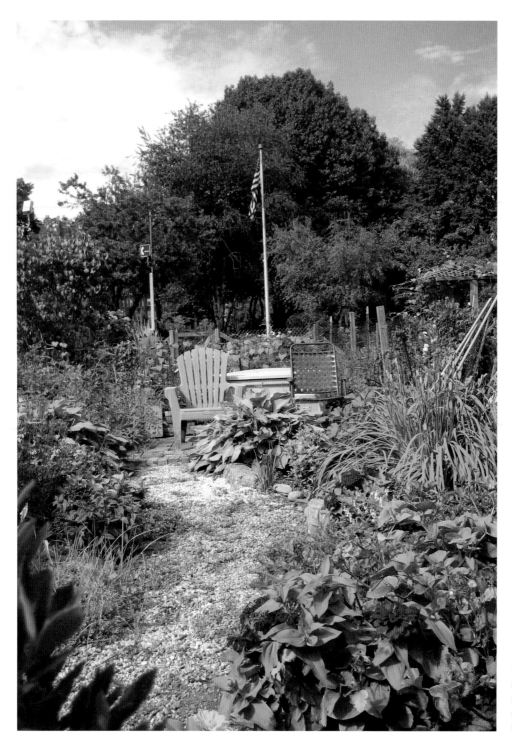

Spirit and patriotism are inexorably entwined in the fabric of the Fenway Victory Gardens in Boston.

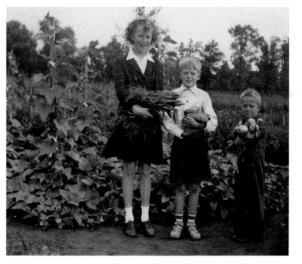

Entire families, including children, cultivated food to "support the troops" at the still-productive Dowling Victory Garden.

with replanting, and little was preserved of the grounds after a parking lot was installed. Sant Pau remained a hospital until 2009; UNESCO is overseeing its restoration as a world heritage site with a museum and cultural center.

Increasingly, social scientists are finding evidence of how the very act of gardening was and is therapeutic, as well as its urgent meaning in times of war. Best known to Americans are the WWII victory allotments in public spaces of highly visible city parks. They were promoted in a national campaign to "support the troops" by producing food needed in a time of war rationing. But they also met broader social and emotional needs by bringing people together in the shared experience of gardening. The Fenway Victory Gardens in Boston have mainly ornamental plants but are still well cared for, as is the Dowling Victory Garden in Minneapolis, which still produces food for the community.

Less well known are stories about the making of gardens in wartime. The therapeutic use of green spaces occurred in the most improbable places, including in the trench gardens carved out by soldiers from the defensive ramparts of WWI. Subsistence gardens were maintained within the walls of the Jewish Ghetto in Warsaw, Poland, during WWII. Traditional Japanese gardens were built and tended by the inhabitants of the internment camps in the western United States during WWII. Soldiers and civilians in Iraq tended and harvested their gardens under constant

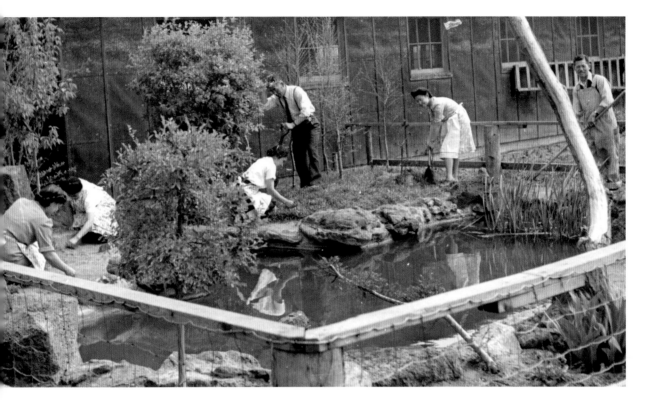

shelling during the recent wars. In these most inhospitable conditions, with threats of violence and death palpable, soldiers, often reputed for hardness and emotional distance, cultivated modest plots of green in a loving and dedicated manner. The motivation was for subsistence but also reconnection to other places and to times of peace and family. As one soldier in Iraq put it, part of it was "just to grow something green out here." And yet, there was an unexpected benefit: the garden helped him cope with missing his family. "I caught myself drifting back to home with the four of us all spending quality family time in our garden" (Helphand 2006).

By cultivating a Japanese garden, internees at the Minidoka "relocation center" were able to connect to their past and escape the present injustice of their incarceration.

Theory

Most people find nature relaxing, and there might be a garden that they know, remember, or imagine that might be especially restorative. That gardens are therapeutic can be proven; the evidence is revealed in research that converges at the intersection of the environment, nature, and health. Most studies are used to advocate for better-designed health-care environments, but their findings are a resource for garden designers in any setting.

"To heal" is defined by Webster's dictionary in three ways: to make sound or whole; to cause (an undesirable condition) to be overcome; to restore to original purity or integrity. In the preamble to its constitution, the World Health Organization defines health as "a state of complete physical, mental, and social well-being and not merely the absence of disease or infirmity." In other words, a distinction must be made between healing and curing. Healing can have physical (albeit not necessarily curative), psychological, and spiritual characteristics. There is a strong relationship between the senses of wholeness (regardless of the trajectory of illness), coherence, and resilience. Those working with distressed communities emphasize the importance of this last especially, equating resilience with finding positive meaning and cultivating positive emotions in times of crisis.

BIOPHILIA

Evolutionary biologist E. O. Wilson (1984) hypothesized that humans have an affinity to other living things; he called this theory biophilia and suggested it was rooted in our biology, in our evolutionary past. Others give a nod to nurture, emphasizing both innate and learned components and recognizing that the tendency to garden is culturally reinforced by watching and helping parents and others with more experience (Kahn and Kellert 2002). While there may be hard-wired connections to the natural world, circumstances and experiences surely shape how each person cultivates them. Readers concerned with children's play and development may recall the book *Last Child in the Woods* (Louv 2005), which identifies a nature-deficit disorder in children and suggests that this deficit might be linked to attention disorders, depression, obesity, and other health conditions.

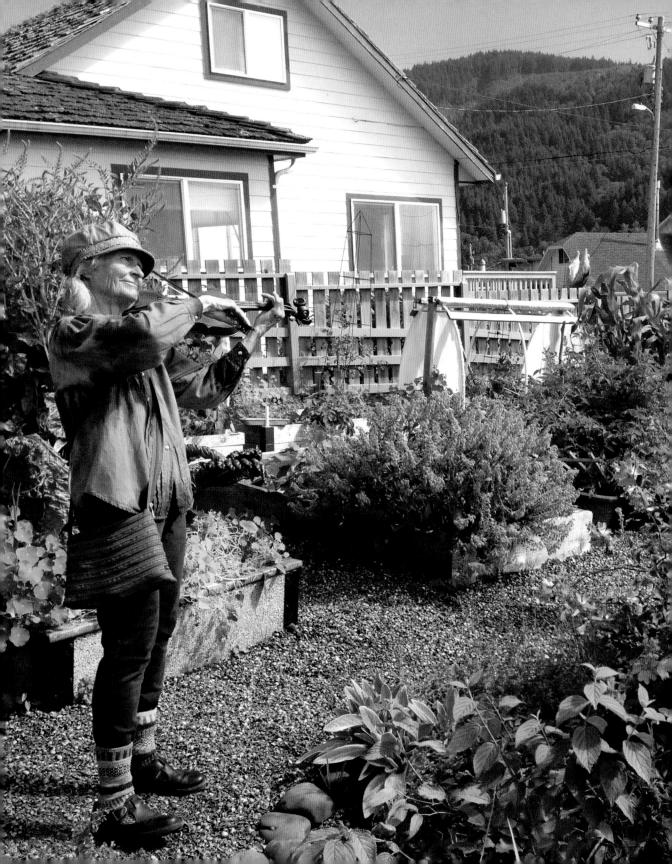

Measurable responses to nature have long been confirmed by research. Behavioral scientist Roger Ulrich (1984) conducted a study of patients recovering from surgery and found those with a view of nature from their hospital window had improved outcomes. By all indications, their vital signs were better; they required less pain medication and had shorter hospital stays. Ulrich and other researchers are continuing to explore psychological and physiological responses to nature and finding factors important to creating therapeutic, healing spaces. This field of inquiry is called evidence-based design and has significant relevance for design and healthcare practitioners.

Stress is identified as the central factor that can both negatively influence health and be mitigated by the environment. Although certain levels of stress stimulate alertness and motivation to act, too much interferes with performance, with coping and recovery, and with a sense of wholeness. In terms of the garden and healing, Ulrich asserts that to mitigate stress people need a sense of control over their surroundings, choices of types of space, opportunities to move and exercise, and to experience positive distractions. Major stressors in healthcare and elder care facilities are lack of privacy, noise, and extremes of light. A supportive garden provides a choice of spaces, varying in enclosure and openness for privacy and social support. Privacy can be found in an open space from which to view and observe others. Spaces for physical movement and exercise are particularly important to the well-being of the elderly, those with or caring for those who are ill, those incarcerated, and children. Consideration for how the spaces are laid out and identified with wayfinding strategies like landmarks will mitigate confusion, another major stressor.

Nature can elevate mood. Nature is among the top four positive distractions that can improve health and well-being, along with comedy/laughter, companion animals, and music. But exactly why nature is restorative is unsettled theory. Ulrich suggests the components are verdant plants, spatial openness with scattered trees, and peaceful wildlife (Ulrich 1991; Ulrich et al. 1991), and subsequent studies have supported that the amount of verdure in the garden is crucial to its restorative qualities (Stigsdotter and Grahn 2002).

Combine music with nature for potent positive distraction. Music is a particular theme in some community gardens.

ATTENTION RESTORATION THEORY

Many of the ideas fundamental to environmental psychologists about the kinds of places people prefer are useful to designing gardens for people coping with stress. Attention Restoration Theory (ART), developed by environmental psychologists Rachel and Stephen Kaplan (1989), highlights the power of natural settings to help people recover from mental fatigue. The focused attention needed to carry out a plan requires effort to push away distractions and leads to fatigue, impulsivity, anger, mistakes, careless behavior, and decreased productivity. Involuntary attention to things that stand out as strange, dynamic, and beautiful is termed fascination. Hard fascination, such as being in a chaotic and busy city, is tiring. Being effortless, soft fascination restores the mind to its vitality and readiness to resume concentration. The natural elements in the garden—plants, birds, wind, clouds—provide soft fascination and elicit a sense of wonder. Further support for restoration in the garden comes from the Kaplans' related concepts of coherence, legibility, complexity, and mystery. People seek coherence in nature or the built environment by looking for and making sense of a pattern in the way things fit together—for example, in the repeating forms of the built elements. They can explore it if they find legibility, understanding they will not get lost or confused. Finally, people will want to discover the garden if it has complexity and mystery—enough variety to be worth learning about and a sense there will be more to unfold than they can predict. People are equally drawn to explore what is new and to return to what they know. They need elements that excite and inspire as well as ones they easily connect with as known and familiar.

Another important concept key to restorative environments is the idea of escape. To offer a sense of getting away, a garden should create another world, a place with soft and quiet fascination to enhance mental wandering. Such a garden would have extent, not in size but in seemingly endless qualities of interest. Sense of depth is primary and can be designed by layers of texture and densities of planting. The blocking of distracting views also enhances the full experience of escape. Designers can use these ideas to think about how users in various states of health will enter the garden and find their way through its spaces with positive experiences of comfort, enrichment, and wonder.

CLOSER LOOK

Thrive

Thrive is a national charity organization based in Reading, England, which champions the benefits of what it calls social and therapeutic horticulture—the process of using gardening, plants, and horticulture to help individuals develop. The group emphasizes nature, health, and a democratic process of community involvement to improve well-being for those with mental, physical, intellectual, and social challenges. The focus of Thrive is to help clients be productive and find a close working relationship with nature. As with those who are changed by gardening through conflict and other times of trauma, clients who participate in Thrive programs emerge with improved resilience and connection to others.

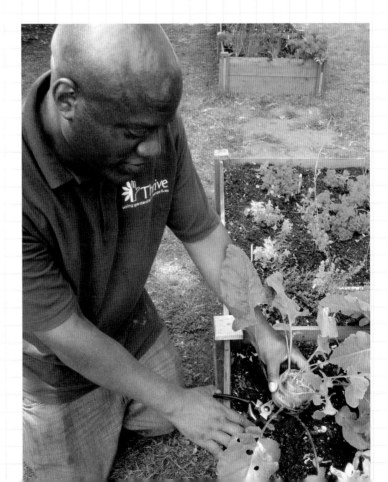

Thrive works with clients at various garden sites in the United Kingdom, "using gardening to change lives."

Applications

Designers use a language of design, their understanding of shaping space, and, for most, an interactive process with their clients to transform the land or rooftop plane into a garden sanctuary. The next chapter covers this in depth, and the book will look at gardens in a range of settings from traditional healthcare institutions and schools to non-traditional settings, grassroots community projects, and gardens for inmates and refugees. Finding that nature itself is restorative, any garden that orchestrates engagement through the senses with nature's pleasing scope and intricacies will offer healing. But users themselves bring a complexity of strengths and needs and ways they engage and respond to a natural setting, and better understanding the people themselves broadens and deepens the healing qualities of the garden. When landscape architects collaborate across disciplines, the benefits are many. Their effective partners when designing therapeutic gardens will be healthcare practitioners and environmental psychologists who understand how people interact with their environments. Incorporating this knowledge in the design deepens the experience of the garden for all—receptivity to different viewpoints is always a catalyst to creative design solutions.

A participatory process is central to designing a therapeutic garden. It reaches out to all interested users, to patients and their care providers, to children and their families, to facility and professional staff. In a series of information-gathering exercises, over one or several meetings, the design team will learn what these people want and expect from the garden they imagine. Potential comforts and activities are often brainstormed as passive and active elements. Designers and therapeutic practitioners together can design, lead, and facilitate this participatory process. Practitioners will relate with empathy and expertise to the strengths and limitations of the users. They will assess all the psychological, social, and physical dimensions at play.

The objectives for the garden will then be assessed and prioritized, measured against universal design (UD) principles and weighed along with user types, site constraints, and costs. The principles of UD are a common ground for problem-solving by designers and therapeutic practitioners; they embrace everyone—those who are ill, those who are

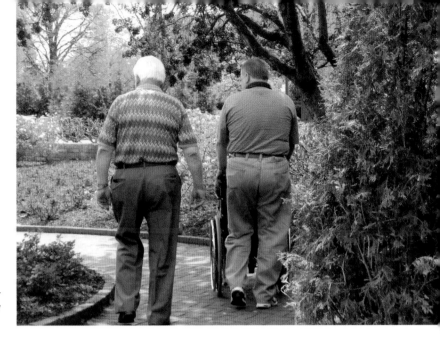

This brick path—smooth, level, and edged with a failsafe "soldier" course—supports UD principles 1, 5, and 6, equitable use, tolerance for error, and low physical effort.

marginalized, those with learning, mental health, mobility, and sensory challenges. Universal design ensures that an environment will be usable by the widest range of users regardless of age, ability, culture, or preference, without further modification. The seven principles are the outcome of research in the built environment and product design, and they are well suited to guiding therapeutic garden design.

1. Equitable use. The garden is appropriate and appealing for all without segregating or stigmatizing users.

2. Flexibility in use. The garden is adaptable to a wide range of individual preferences and abilities and provides choices to accommodate them.

3. Simple and intuitive use. The garden is self-explanatory; there is no excessive energy required to know how and what to do in the space.

4. Perceptible information. The design itself effectively communicates important information regardless of a user's sensory capabilities.

5. Tolerance for error. Features of the garden minimize hazards and the possibility of errors. It provides failsafe features.

6. Low physical effort. The appropriate level of effort is expended to be in and use the garden.

7. Size and space for approach for use. The garden is manageable to be in for all, regardless of body type or mobility status. There are clear lines of sight, reachable components, and adequate space.

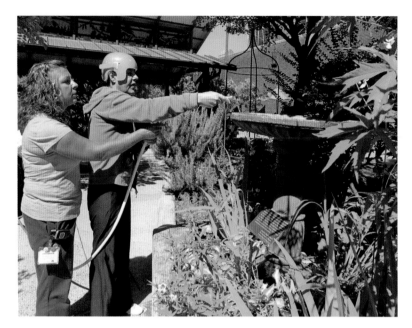

Watering plants as part of an occupational therapy session provides patients the opportunity to engage in a meaningful and purposeful activity.

Universal design is not to be confused with the Americans with Disabilities Act (ADA), which is part of federally mandated design and building code. ADA requires that public buildings and spaces be accessible to people with motor (movement) and visual challenges. It allows older buildings with stepped entries to be retrofitted with ramps but sometimes sacrifices social equity and aesthetic qualities. For example, the slope of an ADA ramp must not exceed 1:12 (that is, every foot of vertical height requires 12 feet of horizontal distance), while the much more gently sloped UD-guided ramp might be 1:20 and fully integrated into the design.

In creating therapeutic gardens for hospitals, elder care centers, and other treatment and community facilities, a transdisciplinary team model is emerging from the healthcare field. It is a collaborative model, in which landscape architects and therapeutic specialists work side-by-side throughout the project. This model of equal partnership goes beyond the traditional one, in which a landscape architectural firm orchestrates and sometimes compartmentalizes the work of designers and engineers. Whatever you call it, trans- or interdisciplinary, this design process marks an exciting departure from standard practice and places the end user at the center of therapeutic garden design.

In the case of therapeutic gardens in care and community facilities, an occupational therapist on the design team brings a particular understanding of human structure, behavior, and function. An occupational therapist helps people do what they want and need to do through the therapeutic use of meaningful and purposeful activity. Occupational therapists serve people of all ages in various settings, from working with infants and their families to meet developmental milestones to supporting adults who have experienced illness or injury to regain function. They are uniquely trained to understand and to adapt environments to support the physical, social, sensory, cognitive, and psychological needs associated with a wide range of disease and disability. Most relevant to garden design, they understand how to remove barriers to participation and how to choose, organize, and adapt features of the environment to fit people.

An occupational therapist on the design team will continually evaluate how the users interact with the garden elements. An environmental psychologist will evaluate the therapeutic benefits in terms of the emotional and perceptual responses that people will have with the garden. When the garden includes therapy programs, it may also be beneficial to partner with affiliated practitioners, such as physical, speech, recreational, horticultural, and music therapists, social workers, and clinical psychologists. There may be formal treatments and group activities that can be conducted outside in the garden's natural setting or with integrated therapeutic elements. The therapists say what garden elements are needed. For example, at the recommendation of the physical or occupational therapist, a path might be equipped with railings at various heights, stairs and ramps with distinct levels of ambulation challenge, rings and bars for upper body strengthening and conditioning, and wayfinding elements for those with visual impairment to develop the confidence and skills needed to work on orientation and mobility skills. Activities can range from active exercises to more passive therapist-designed reflections, including journal writing, breathing exercises, and sensory pathways to meditation.

In most gardens, the gardening itself will be the purposeful and meaningful work that relieves stress and restores confidence and well-being. Depending on the organizational structure, a gardening program may be guided by a recreational, occupational, or horticultural therapist. The American Horticultural Therapy Association (AHTA) defines a therapeutic garden as a "plant-dominated environment purposefully designed to facilitate interaction with healing elements of nature"; the association

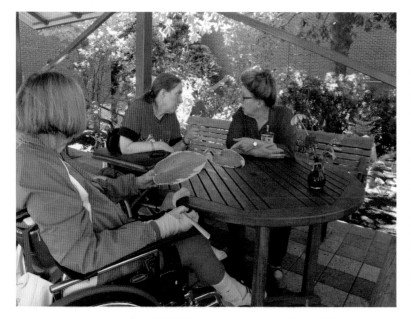

TOP Teresia Hazen, coordinator of therapeutic gardens and horticultural therapy at Legacy Health in Portland, Oregon, meets with clients in a garden she helped design.

BOTTOM A speech therapy session conducted in a garden, where there is much to talk about, can inspire both patient and therapist.

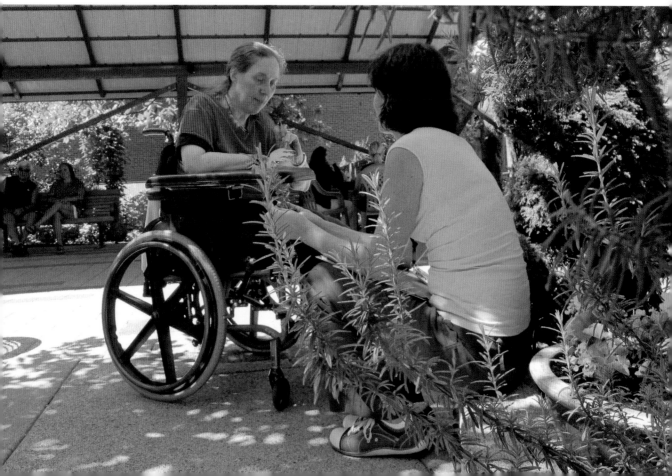

has identified seven common characteristics likely to be associated with excellence in the design of therapeutic gardens: scheduled and pro-grammed activities; features modified to improve accessibility; well-defined perimeters; a profusion of plants and people/plant interactions; benign and supportive conditions; universal design; and recognizable placemaking.

An integral part of designing for clients is to offer care providers some guidance on how to get the most out of the therapeutic garden. User and informational manuals, video guides, maps, and signage will help all therapists, whether staff or consultants, maximize the garden's benefits as a therapy tool. The occupational therapist can include recommended activities, as well as ways to make them easier or harder for patients. The manual may have visuals showing the intended use of such elements as parallel bars, accessible swings, raised beds, and workout stations. A video can provide a guided tour of the garden and hands-on demon-strations of how every element is operated; it can also address potential safety concerns, including whether certain elements are to be used only under a therapist's supervision.

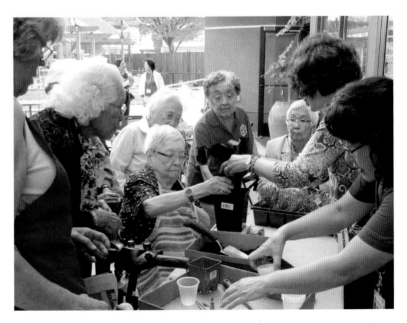

An "up-potting" session is a great way to bring a group of people together with a common purpose.

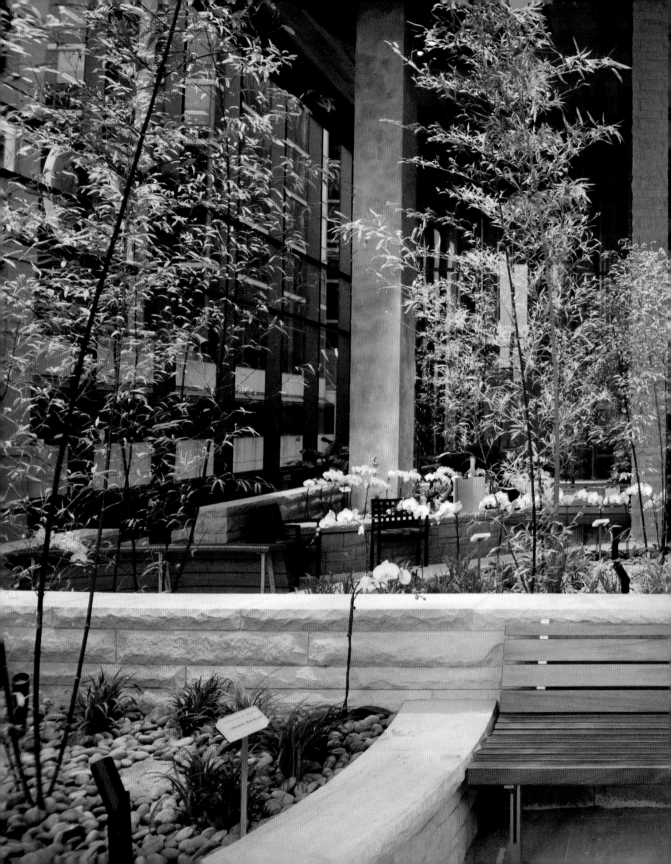

CHAPTER TWO
COLLABORATIVE DESIGN

Design is a collaborative process that unfolds in a sequence of phases, from initial project goals to final design and construction plans. In this chapter the process will be described as it is led by a design team of landscape architect and occupational therapist, partnering to make therapeutic gardens; both commit to the idea that design is a participatory process, and the therapeutic benefits of the garden are built by keeping the team's focus on the clients or users. Following the sections on design sequence is a discussion of major design elements: grading, rooms, paths, and plants. Throughout, the team uses a framework of four principles that will infuse their design with therapeutic values and benefits (Ulrich 1991).

1. Sense of control (actual and perceived). The garden allows individuals to make choices. It provides a temporary escape, a sensation of "being away," an opportunity for the user to gain control of his or her emotions and refocus attention.

2. Sense of belonging and connection. The garden has familiarity and fosters a sense of attachment and place. It has a variety of enclosed and public spaces for private and open exchanges.

3. Movement and exercise. The garden supports low-impact activities, including walking, wheeled mobility, gardening, play, formal exercise, and physical rehabilitation. These activities build strength, reduce stress, and elevate mood.

4. Sensory nourishment. The garden offers heightened interactions with nature through the senses. Natural distractions improve emotional states, diminish troublesome thoughts, and foster positive physiological outcomes.

Shared by an occupational therapist: I worked at a continuing-care retirement community that received a grant to install a vegetable garden. The plan was more or less that the residents would work in the garden with help from the Big Brothers and Big Sisters participants who came to visit regularly. The veggies would be used by dining services for the residents' meals. I know that no one in the therapy department was consulted in the design of the gardens. They put in four or five long rectangular raised beds, just six to eight inches above the ground, with the beds on a fairly steep slope and grass paths around them. The design of the beds guaranteed that no one using a wheelchair would be able to get near the beds since they couldn't get the chairs up the steep grass slope. There weren't any chairs or benches nearby, so people who walked a fair distance to get there weren't able to rest before heading back.

Once the garden was built, the therapy department was asked to use the garden as part of our treatment plans. I would occasionally take people there just to get them some fresh air, but none of my residents were able to actually work in the garden the way it was designed. I never saw any of the residents, even the independent-living folks, working in the garden or even spending much time there. It was neglected pretty much from the beginning. I'm not sure whether there was a water source located close to the garden or whether they were planning for the sprinkler system to handle the watering, but I don't think there was a plan in place for regular watering, and in the Texas summer, the garden needed daily attention to thrive. A few months after the garden was installed, all the plants had withered. It was such a sad story because so many of the residents were interested in gardening, and the therapists were excited about using the garden, but it was designed in such a way that it made it very difficult for the majority of the residents to even sit and look at it, much less do any actual planting or maintenance. I think this is a perfect example of an opportunity wasted, as well as an example of how good intentions made the situation worse, as having the dead garden visible for everyone to see was infinitely more depressing than not having a garden at all.

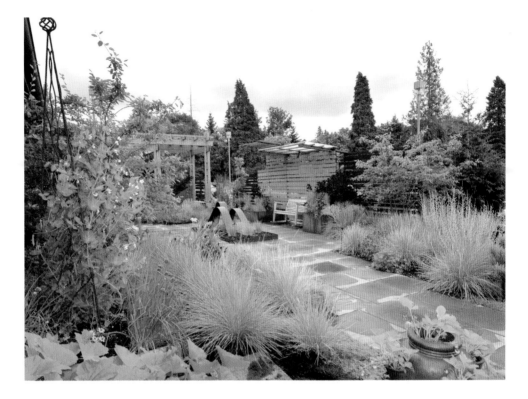

Therapeutic gardens designed with the four principles in mind offer a wide range of therapeutic value for users.

When the designer and therapist work collaboratively and with flexibility, the design solutions tend to be meaningful and appropriate. A garden with therapeutic benefits will have both universal qualities and those that respond specifically to the complexity of needs people have for restoration. For users, the garden is a counterpoint to a confining environment and regimen that, while it supports their recovery or well-being, may not relieve their stress. Based on evidence that just being in nature positively affects health, the garden that immerses users in an enhanced experience of nature through all the senses is a place for healing.

The objective for most therapeutic gardens is to provide opportunities for restoration, movement, play, and exercise, and often for integrated therapy programs. When users are deprived of a sense of free agency or control, a garden that offers them choices and levels of accessibility supports their engagement and confidence. When the qualities and elements of the garden express and reinforce the user's sense of familiarity and cultural attachment, they feel a sense of comfort and belonging. The designer looks to balance familiarity with mystery and wonder in the process of orchestrating the grading, rooms, paths, and plants of the garden in a coherent manner.

Understanding Goals

The proposal for a therapeutic garden project originates as a set of goals shaped by a design advisory committee before they hire the design team. The committee will have a site and a preliminary idea of the project's scope and budget. The design team collaborates with the design advisory committee to refine and prioritize the project goals. Sometimes objectives need shaping for feasibility, and a brainstorming session can be helpful to explore alternatives for specific purposes. Ideally the advisory committee includes the broadest range of stakeholders—a staff specialist, a patient, a physical plant manager, and an administrator, at a minimum. The design team will learn about the community from their different points of view and begin to understand health conditions, therapy programs, desired outcomes, access, safety, and maintenance concerns. The process can be challenging, but ideally, through discussion and compromise, consensus is achieved. If not, there are other ways of driving decisions forward. If the number of advisory members is odd, not even, one option is majority vote, or the designer arbitrates to resolve differences. Once the goals have been developed and needs expressed, they are clustered around themes—for example, short- and long-term objectives, patient or resident and staff concerns, and problems to be addressed.

Participatory Design

The best way for a designer to understand user needs is to encourage all stakeholders to participate; their responses are vital and will inform the design process. Including users in the creative process illuminates the range and specificity of their needs and, crucially, is a key to developing stewardship for the garden once it is completed. Rooted in Scandinavia and emerging in the 1960s and '70s, participatory design was originally a means of addressing early-stage design issues. The process typically begins with a series of informational sessions with existing and potential users. Patients, residents, staff, administrators, visitors, and family members share their viewpoints and preferences in a series of prepared exercises. Participatory design is inclusive, accessible to all participants regardless of their age, status, or abilities. Innovative methods that align with specific projects may need to be developed to bridge differences of language, socio-economic and cultural background, physical abilities, cognition, and education.

RESPECTFULLY ENGAGING ALL USERS
Using terms such as "people with disabilities" instead of "disabled person" acknowledges that they are people first, and not a disability. Words like "handicapped" and "retarded" are derogatory and offensive, and may cause harm. Identifying someone as a cancer "victim" or an arthritis "sufferer" implies that the person's quality of life is diminished. A disability should never define a person.

Impairment is the loss or abnormality of a body part, or some type of mental dysfunction. A person who has had a spinal cord injury and cannot move his or her legs is impaired. A disability is something a person cannot do because of an impairment. This same person who cannot walk because of the spinal cord injury has a disability. A handicap is a limiting factor imposed on someone by environmental conditions or other people's actions. A disability can become a handicap for the person with a spinal cord injury if the slope of a wheelchair ramp is too steep or a pathway is too uneven to navigate safely.

PARTICIPATORY DESIGN IN GUATEMALA CITY

In 2007, a landscape architecture design/build team was invited to Guatemala City to create a series of therapeutic gardens at an educational facility for families supporting themselves by working in the largest garbage dump in Central America. The families subsist by scavenging and selling recyclable materials. Most were displaced from their Mayan highland villages by the 30-year civil war, and many speak an indigenous Mayan dialect. Most were uncomfortable expressing their ideas to outsiders in group meetings, but through trial and error, the design team discovered that the mothers and children responded enthusiastically to photo-preference exercises. Being sensitive to attendee needs, these and other visual methods were implemented instead of speaking at length through a translator. Participants expressed their preferences by ranking images related to learning and play activities, social gathering, and aesthetic qualities. They attached green and red stickers to the images to indicate their likes and dislikes, respectively.

To explore their ideas in form and space, they created paper collages and models in clay and cardboard. Tagging images in books was also effective with the children and adults. These particular exercises, oral

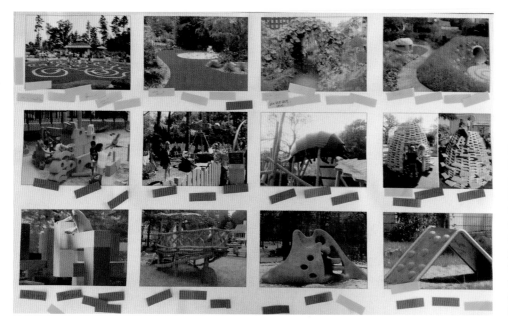

Indicating preferences for design elements with stickers, green for yes and red for no (or smile or frown stickers), is a simple and effective way to garner information from the community when language or other communication barriers exist.

surveys, and brainstorming sessions were facilitated using translators. The design team analyzed the entire pattern of their needs and preferences. They preferred highly colorful plants and abundant nature not found in their current living situation but which reminded them of home. They also wanted gender-neutral play opportunities, age separation for the preschool children, and safety for all.

PARTICIPATORY DESIGN AT NIKKEI MANOR

In 2012, a design team began work with elderly Japanese Americans to create a courtyard garden for their senior care residence, Nikkei Manor, in Seattle. Many of the residents did not speak English or found focusing in active group settings with loud talking too distracting. The team developed a card game to understand their preferences. In one-on-one meetings, resident participants were given a deck of cards with garden images printed on them. Each was asked to sort the cards into two piles, one for likes and one for dislikes. The game-like quality was appealing, and the directness of the exercise was compatible with variable levels of abilities and comprehension. Meeting one-on-one opened up the opportunity for a simple discussion between the participant and the design team member.

Often this method clarified why the residents chose certain images. In several cases very personal stories emerged that told of their past and of what they imagined the garden to be, things they might not have been comfortable sharing in a large-group activity. Many spoke fondly of the traditional Japanese rock and moss gardens of their childhood and felt they wanted this archetypal garden at Nikkei Manor. In the card game, residents selected images of colorful gardens, with abundant seasonal bloom, lush foliage, and texture. The design team and advisory committee discussed the expertise required to create a traditional garden that contained diverse religious symbolism, and arrived at a Pacific Northwest interpretation of a Japanese garden. From discussion with staff, the design team learned that the transition from home to assisted living is disorienting for many older adults. Many residents experience apprehension, depression, confusion, and loneliness during the transition from independent living and productivity to a group living situation. Loss of independence, work, or avocation can mean loss of identity. The garden can ease this transition and remind residents of home.

An informed written summary of the findings from these types of exercises, surveys, and meetings with participants is next presented to and discussed with the design advisory committee. The designers respond to all they learned about the community when they begin to design the garden, including cultural backgrounds, familiar place attachments, and specific health conditions. By working with an occupational therapist, designers have an increased awareness of health conditions and users' strengths and weaknesses. The summary lists programmatic activities, with some indication of how these will be apportioned among the various spaces from which users can choose (quiet and enclosed, active and open). The designers use this information to choose elements, forms, and expressions users will respond to in the garden.

To expand gardening capacities at Nikkei Manor, grant funding was later provided to design and install a vertical garden for the second-floor balcony, located just off the dining room. Again working as a team from the outset, the occupational therapist and landscape designer and several other staff and volunteers led 41 residents and staff members through a three-station activity. The entire participatory design process took place in the courtyard garden of the facility, which by then had been installed by a University of Washington landscape architecture design/build studio class. One activity station had two card-sorts and an age-range identifier task; the purpose was to inform the garden's look and planting theme. Two other stations looked at four different anthropometric measures to determine the garden's specifications and dimensions for optimal usability by the widest range of users, as some of the residents used canes or walkers to help with ambulation. All 41 participants completed the activities at the three stations. A second community meeting was held to get feedback on a half-scale model of the proposed vertical garden. The group of about 25 residents and day care attendees overwhelmingly approved it (and even got their hands dirty, potting up individual cells of the garden). From a seated or standing position, the garden was comfortable for all.

Sorting images into likes and dislikes eliminates the need for words, and often, as with other card games, sparks conversation and stimulates memories.

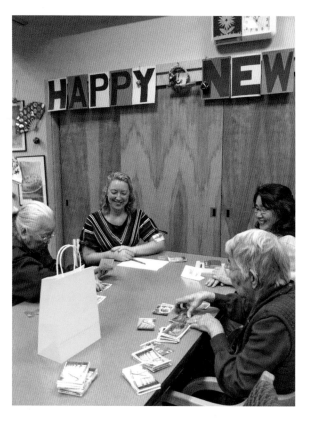

Site Assessment

The design team begins its assessment of a site's inherent opportunities and constraints with a wide view of the site's context: they study maps and aerial and satellite photographs to learn how the site relates to existing circulation routes, open space patterns, forested areas, and housing densities. Designers need to know the site's dimensions, its topography, and the exact location of fixed elements. Municipal plot plans will show property boundaries and existing buildings and parking areas, but a scaled professional survey is the most accurate and thorough documentation of existing site conditions. The client sometimes provides it; alternatively, a licensed surveyor is contracted to prepare one using GPS and/or laser surveying equipment. The survey shows, at scale and with legally binding accuracy, property boundaries, topography, paved surfaces, walls, buildings, trees, shrubs, and water features. This information determines the carrying capacity of the site. Access points and existing adjacent uses are identified, including entries, waiting rooms, dining areas, or rehabilitation clinics. The designers start to think about how to connect these activity areas to the garden, to its plantings and arbors, to its paths or rooms, to its private and open spaces. If patient or resident rooms look into the site, this is noted for later decisions about enhancing or screening views. The compatibility of existing uses will strongly influence design solutions. The process of assessing a roof deck, which has weight load and other more specific concerns, is covered in a later section.

Information on grades, drainage, soils, and the location of utilities is also determinative. A locator service for the utility companies identifies and marks the location of underground utilities, which could be disrupted by excavation in the garden's construction and will need to be accessed for ongoing maintenance. Measures of the site's slopes or grades will inform the design of accessible paths and open spaces and influence which planting areas will be retained and where structures and ramps will be incorporated. Soil conditions are available from county records, but most designers take soil samples for testing at a local lab. Some soils like compacted clay are challenging to improve even if amended, and plants may need a different location or a raised bed. Soil tests will also indicate any heavy metals, such as lead, retained by the soils if the site had prior industrial uses or proximity to older structures with sloughing lead paint; such soils are unsafe for gardening activities.

The survey, aerial images, and plot plans do not convey essential qualitative sensory information, such as light and wind patterns, sounds, scents, color, materiality, the flows and rhythms of movement, or pleasing views. Additionally, photographs are taken of welcome and undesirable views that the designers will try to enhance or block out, respectively. All these sensory qualities will resonate with the therapeutic aspects of the garden. It is invaluable to spend time on the site to walk, sit, observe, sketch, listen, and experience these qualities to understand the phenomenological character of what the site is and might become.

Site evaluation includes considering what elements may be challenging for users and what changes will increase universal access and use. If the population includes those with visual impairments, the team should evaluate the light quality and contrasting shadow patterns to decide if additional lighting must be employed or vegetation removed. The team assesses existing landmarks: are they successful wayfinding cues, or will additional features be required to assist with orientation, wayfinding, and directionality? The team should consider whether the site can be comfortably experienced through a single path for those with mobility challenges, or whether multiple loop paths would better accommodate a range of abilities.

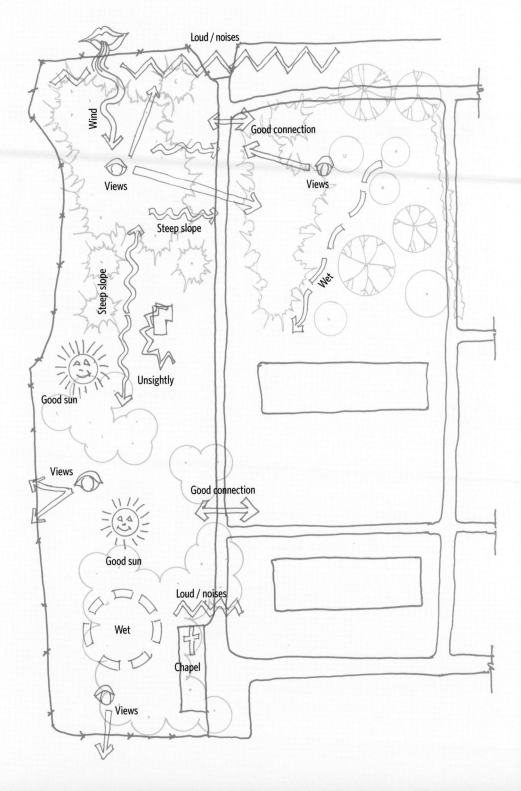

In order to capitalize on positive features and to mediate unsightly objects, undesirable views, unwanted sounds, or dangerous conditions, designers must first spend significant time on site.

Loud / noises

Wind

Good connection

Views

Views

Steep slope

Steep slope

Unsightly

Good sun

Views

Good connection

Wet

Good sun

Loud / noises

Wet

Chapel

Views

Conceptual Design

In the next phase, designers generate multiple options for organizing elements and activities on the garden site into three to four conceptual designs. In conceptualizing, activities and programs are drawn and labeled as simple bubble diagrams on the site plan, so the designers can consider how they will spatially and functionally relate to one another and to adjacent uses. The garden needs to have good circulation and flow if people are to intuitively understand how to move about its spaces.

Often, user preferences from participatory design add up to more than the site can accommodate. In the bubble diagrams, designers prioritize them in various ways and try to place multiple functions in one space. The diagrams articulate at rough scale areas of use such as gathering tables, meditation paths, performance space, edible garden. Designers usually find multiple ways to orient them on the site, allowing the client to compare their merits and respond.

The designers analyze all the opportunities and constraints of the site as learned in the site assessment. An overlay to the site plan notes these as specific attributes. Steep slopes, for example, are shown in the overlay, as they orient to accessible paths and activities. Significant fixed elements are marked as assets to be preserved or enhanced, such as mature trees or beautiful views or advantageous areas for planting beds. Others such as utilities are noted for moving or screening or, if underground, as caution areas. Views that are unwanted or problematic are marked for visual screening. Sun, shade, and soil conditions are specifically noted: they may negatively impact certain activities and users, such as those who are photosensitive or immune-compromised. All the observed phenomena of the site—whether concrete, such as historic remnants, or qualities, such as quiet, mysterious, escape, reflective, aromatic—are summarized and located on the overlay.

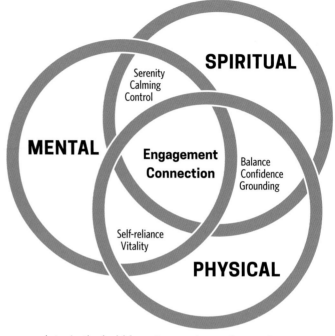

SPIRITUAL

Serenity
Calming
Control

MENTAL

Engagement Connection

Balance
Confidence
Grounding

Self-reliance
Vitality

PHYSICAL

A concept diagram illustrates the broad abstract ideas that will guide the design.

A concept diagram
locating activities.

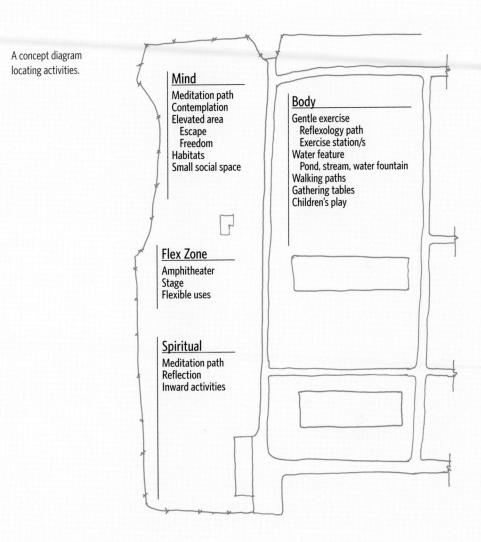

Mind

Meditation path
Contemplation
Elevated area
  Escape
  Freedom
Habitats
Small social space

Flex Zone

Amphitheater
Stage
Flexible uses

Spiritual

Meditation path
Reflection
Inward activities

Body

Gentle exercise
  Reflexology path
  Exercise station/s
Water feature
  Pond, stream, water fountain
Walking paths
Gathering tables
Children's play

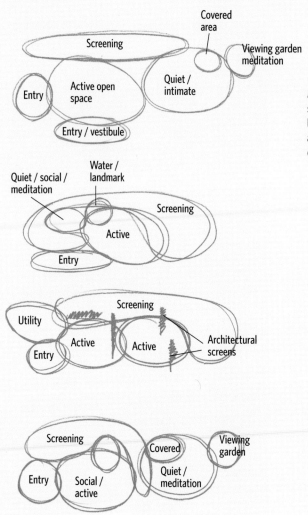

A bubble diagram, representing scale and sequence in a proposed garden. The relationship between the activities, their location in space, and their size become the foundations for the design.

CONCEPTUAL DESIGN AT NIKKEI MANOR

The conceptual design process used at Nikkei Manor shows how the findings from the participatory process together with the site analysis generate design ideas. Three layers of drawings were assembled: the site base plan, a site analysis overlay, and one each of four different design concept overlays. The site base plan provided by Nikkei as a survey showed the site's long, narrow, and flat wedge-like shape. At its longest boundary was a retaining wall, 60 feet long by 30 inches high, with a two-story warehouse behind. Opposite was the east side of the three-story residence. The angular short sides were fenced for security. At one end, along an arterial, was a 12-inch-high stepped egress; at the other end were the utilities and a gate to the parking lot. Two old cherry trees were remnants of a previous garden. Large water tanks for disaster preparedness sat in an open area. Two doors opened to the garden, one for residents and one for a staff lounge room. The site's concrete slab was demolished, and new slabs were installed.

The site analysis overlay suggested where improvements and enhancements were needed. The blank wall of the warehouse was a bleak, looming presence and needed screening. The retaining wall in front was the remnant of a memorable historic hotel—a value worth retaining. At the arterial end the traffic was noisy, but this area received the most sun and had a small garden. A landmark and screening was necessary to bring people into this part of the site. The emergency egress was not ADA accessible. One of the cherry trees was in poor shape, but the other was stately and beloved by the residents. The mechanicals and water tanks were eyesores. The fences and gate to the parking were of medium height and poor quality. Resident rooms did not face the garden because the upper story windows were aligned with corridors. The glass wall of the staff room viewed the garden. The access door for residents was solid and at the end of a long, dark passageway. A request was made for a glass replacement door, and the overlay noted the need for a landmark aligned by sight from the passageway. Finally, the gate entry was kept locked, opened only for public occasions.

Four different design concept overlays were made, all adhering to the client's prevailing idea to have open sightlines throughout the garden. Each design assigned space for an array of the many activities and elements requested by users. Each layout diagrammed one, two, or three rooms for multiple uses. All the designs programmed flexible active spaces for craft classes, celebrations, outdoor eating, games, pet programs, and exercises. As requested, this open space accommodated five movable round tables and chairs to seat 30 people. Two of the concept designs had a quiet, more removed space that could be both a stage for music and performances and a private retreat for reading, rest, meditation, tea ceremonies, and spiritual focus. The gated entries varied in size and orientation. Two concepts included a covered area, one a water fountain, and two a single ramp to a raised deck. They had differing concepts of where to elevate parts of the site and where to locate plants and seating and where to provide screening. They made varying use of landmarks, but all preserved the healthy cherry tree.

Schematic Design

In schematic design, the designer represents at scale and in three dimensions the garden elements indicated by the conceptual design diagrams. The process is exploratory, with the goal being to find the best design and coordination of paths, plazas, planting beds, play elements, seating, structures, and other specified features. The designer locates them and defines their form and material qualities. Each of the conceptual designs is pushed to a solution that is comprehensible, accessible, nurturing, and feasible, generating many ideas that clients can compare and evaluate. The final design is usually a synthesis, a new refinement, of multiple options from the schematics.

The following are some of the challenges designers will face at this phase, depending on client objectives, user needs and preferences, and site conditions.

• How will nature infuse the garden?

• How will the activities be layered to fit the carrying capacity of the site?

• How can the garden layout be clear and coherent while offering users appropriate levels of choice and complexity?

• How much space will be allocated to paths to grade and size them for universal access and to offer both escape and connection?

• How will landmarks be incorporated or designed to orient users?

• How will the primary and secondary entries be differentiated to be identifiable and transition the visitor to and from the garden?

• How will contiguous existing and designed spaces and their activities relate to each other in their separation, sequencing, and flow? Do they offer compatible experiences?

• How can each space be differentiated, shaped, and sized to support the activities designated to it?

• How will choices the garden offers be appropriate for each user's given capacity and need for control?

- How can pleasing sights and sounds in and near the garden be shaped and enhanced? How will the unappealing views and noises be screened and masked?

- How can rehabilitation challenges and opportunities be integrated into the garden?

- How can the garden provide cultural familiarity in the selection of types of plants? In the colors, patterns, and motifs of built structures?

- How can hands-on growing opportunities be integrated to engage the broadest range of gardeners?

In the schematic designs, the design solutions are now tested and adjusted by representing the elements in plan and section drawings. Plan drawings show overhead views of how all the site elements are laid out. They will show, for example, the depth and width (not the height) of an entry arbor and how it connects to a path. Section drawings are made to show grade changes throughout the site. The sections allow designers to consider the elements at their height and in a horizontal view they choose. A view might show the relative heights of people to fences, trees, and slopes. A section is needed to evaluate the extent of a ramp as it relates to an overhead pergola. Designers use both types of drawings to explore materials and patterns; they evaluate the paving patterns for a plaza, the geometries of structures built of wood, or designs for fountains. Plants are indicated on these drawings by their types, arrangement, and massing. Simple three-dimensional computer images and models using cardboard, clay, and wood show the massing of forms on the entire site.

When the designers resolve each of the schematic designs, they construct a proposal for each option. In a meeting with the design advisory committee and interested community members, they narrate the merits of each design, using drawings, illustrative models, and computer animations. Usually each of the options will meet most of the objectives in some way and with different emphasis. The designers will try to synthesize the best components of each design into their final proposal. The proposals are often then posted on a website for wider community input.

SCHEMATIC DESIGN AT NIKKEI MANOR

The designers of the therapeutic garden at Nikkei Manor brought their four schematic designs to the design advisory committee for discussion.

The advisors compared the layouts and preferred plan A: sightlines were clear throughout, and the two spaces, though defined as separate, appeared to flow together. All the plans had a ramp to the emergency egress to meet ADA code. Plans A and D also saw this 12-inch-high grade change at the street as an opportunity to raise this entire end of the site. The modest vertical separation of the deck created a sense of escape, and the covered pavilion there became a destination. Behind it, the sunken viewing garden offered both a surprising discovery and cultural familiarity. This viewing garden was a traditional dry rock garden with a statue of Buddha.

Looking at the four plazas, the advisors liked the concrete pattern of plan C. They felt the residents would respond to how the joints were scored to appear like tatami mats. Plans B and D had water features placed directly opposite the resident entry, which would be a helpful landmark to orient users, especially if the water was made audible to those with visual impairments.

At the public entry, reviewers preferred the wide arbor at the opening into the garden shown by plan C. They also liked the gateway panels that staggered and flanked the entry in plan D. Plan C also effectively moved the water tanks to a corner near the utilities. A new high fence was placed to hide them, and its design and ornamentation connected to the entry arbor in a strong linear sequence. These ideas combined could make this secured entrance a welcoming place for visitors and an identifiable presence in the neighborhood.

All plans prominently featured the remaining cherry tree and put seating there, and all used a sequence of plants to screen the warehouse wall. Advisors responded positively to the opportunities each scheme found to use planters to mark entries or to surround the seating. Soft enclosure and incorporation of sensory-rich plantings would support the primary activities of thoughtful retreat and observation, walking, and mental wandering. The cornered seat nooks featured in plans B and C would promote conversation.

The separate plaza and deck of plans A and D has the greatest potential benefit for Nikkei's regular social, recreational, and therapeutic programming. Each space was flexible as to seating arrangements (including no seating, to allow for movement). The deck and plaza had enough separation to be used concurrently, and the two spaces could function together as a performance stage and audience seating.

While there were places to walk to in each scheme, only A and D, by including a ramp, referenced a path. In studying the schemes together, a new idea emerged to place a second ramp under the pergola extending from the pavilion in plan A. This effectively created a loop walking path, ascending to and descending from the deck. The loop path greatly improved circulation in the garden and introduced a new universally accessible therapeutic benefit.

Design Development

When the design advisory committee has reviewed the schematic designs, their input is analyzed and the design development phase begins. In this process of synthesis and refinement, the design team brings together the preferred elements from each of the schematic designs. The designers render each element to its precise dimensions, showing the materials used and resolving every functional and aesthetic detail. The planting plan now lists the taxa required and their quantities, and illustrates where to locate the species and cultivars in planters and beds. The goals are to refine the design to a level of constructability, to meet all code and permitting requirements, and to be within budget. The design phase concludes with construction documentation, consisting of a construction drawing set and a project manual with specifications for building. The plan, section, and elevation drawings are computer-drafted for accuracy and for easily making changes. This information is used by the contractor to bid and build the project. Construction begins when a contractor is chosen and contracts are signed.

The design team's involvement continues through the building process. The lead consultant assumes the role of project manager and stays in contact with the client, attending project meetings, monitoring the budget, and responding to requests for information, clarifications, or changes in the design. Other team members are included in the process to answer questions and review submittals pertinent to their expertise.

DESIGN DEVELOPMENT AT NIKKEI MANOR

In this last phase, a second ramp was added linking the plaza and the deck at the outer wall. In the long perpendicular space between the ramps, designers detailed a poured concrete planter large enough for a red-leaved Japanese maple and mounds of red- and pink-flowering azaleas. Corner benches of wood with curved steel arm supports bordered the planters on either side of both deck and plaza. Ramps were sloped at 1:20 and surfaced with plastic lumber with a skid-resistant texture; the designers integrated kick rails and black metal handrails. At a generous five feet in width, the ramps appeared to flow from the plaza plane. The cohesive connection of the spaces was enhanced by echoing the tatami mat pattern of the concrete plaza in the orientation of the wood decking.

The final design development drawing for Nikkei Manor's Ichi-go Icho-e courtyard garden illustrates the location, size, and scale of all proposed elements. Planting, paving patterns, and materials are fully rendered, and callouts clarify the kind of spaces and features being proposed.

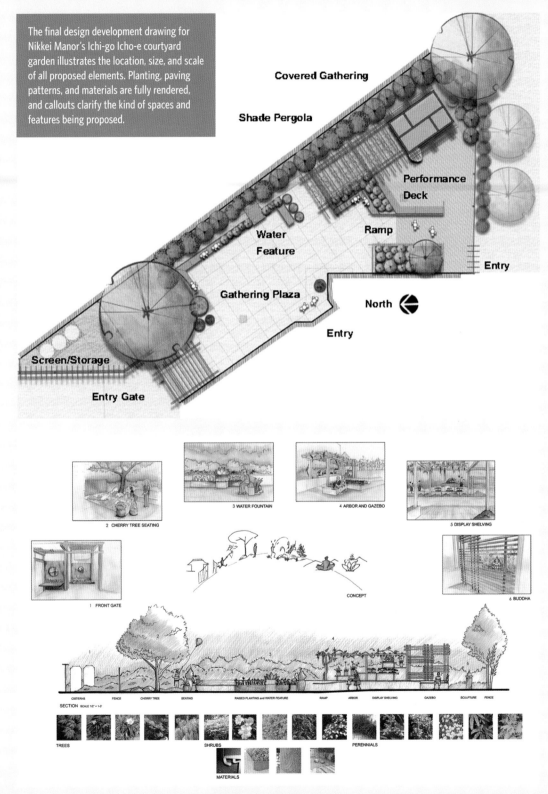

Covered Gathering

Shade Pergola

Performance Deck

Ramp

Water Feature

Entry

Gathering Plaza

North

Screen/Storage

Entry

Entry Gate

2 CHERRY TREE SEATING

3 WATER FOUNTAIN

4 ARBOR AND GAZEBO

5 DISPLAY SHELVING

1 FRONT GATE

CONCEPT

6 BUDDHA

CISTERNS   FENCE   CHERRY TREE   SEATING   RAISED PLANTING and WATER FEATURE   RAMP   ARBOR   DISPLAY SHELVING   GAZEBO   SCULPTURE   FENCE

SECTION SCALE 1/2" = 1'-0"

TREES

SHRUBS

PERENNIALS

MATERIALS

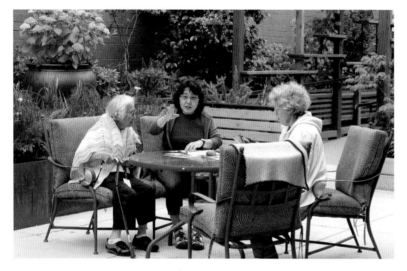

TOP Seating that meets the needs of the intended user group enhances the likelihood that a garden will be used. Armrests on chairs and benches make it easier for older adults to sit down and rise.

BOTTOM Universal design features like a low sloping ramp, plant shelves at varied heights, and integrated railings exponentially increase the inclusivity of the garden for the Nikkei community.

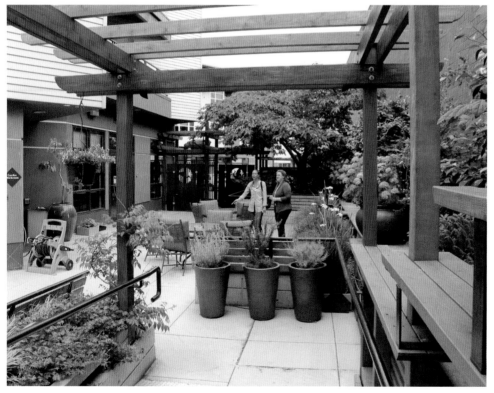

The loop path would offer gentle exercise and a companionable journey, and planted seating areas would be readily available everywhere along the route. On the outer wall along the second ramp, shelving at different heights was fitted to the trellis structure; here, residents could seasonally display and care for their bonsai and other houseplants.

A pattern of alternating steel planters and custom wood benches wrapped around the plaza. Plants were abundantly layered under the cherry tree and along the entire length of the retaining wall. Hydrangeas, camellias, and Leyland cypress screened the warehouse façade at the top of the wall. Between the planters at the base of the wall, just opposite the entry door, the water fountain was placed to become a wayfinding landmark. The steel-panel fountain, five and a half feet in height, was pierced with three slotted scuppers dropping water into three bowls filled with amber glass. At the fountain's head was a large stylized lotus blossom with one of the scuppers at its base, so the stream of water resembled its stem. The sound of falling and splashing water would indeed be audible from the residence entry door.

The design team focused on making the pavilion both a landmark and a destination that would be experienced as a semi-private retreat. For those seeking exercise, it is also the midpoint in a loop up and down the adjacent ramps. The pavilion connected to the trellis and was tied visually to all the wood built structures, using the same bypass framing, similarly sized lumber, and a color scheme of red, black, and yellow. It had the same detailing of rafter ends as the entry arbor, overall expressing a traditional Japanese approach to design. The pavilion was covered with polycarbonate panels, tinted a smoke color to reduce glare. Movable cushioned seating would be available year-round. A window opening in the pavilion wall was oriented to a hidden sunken garden for contemplation.

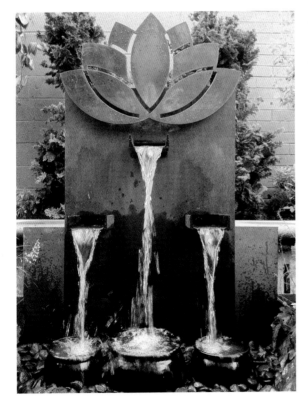

This water feature functions as a wayfinding element. Located directly opposite the interior glass door leading out to the garden, residents see and hear it as they approach.

A katsura tree was planted at this corner of the site. Also at street side, along the whole length of the deck, the fence was softened and buffered by a 14-foot hedge of fargesia, a non-invasive bamboo.

In response to the design advisory committee, the team decided the entry gate should both further heighten the sense of passage for the visitor and mark the garden's presence in the neighborhood. From site corner to building corner, they created a sequence of fencing, gateway, and pergola, repeating the traditional Japanese design language of the deck structures. At the gate the visitor would enter, turning to their left between ornamental steel panels, first glimpsing the garden through one and then another of the panel's round cutouts. A crane motif animates the garden:

The exterior entry features a sheltered bench and a threshold with a change in pavement—a visual and tactile alert for visitors to understand they are entering the garden. The Ichi-go Ichi-e sign is modeled on traditional forms found in Japan.

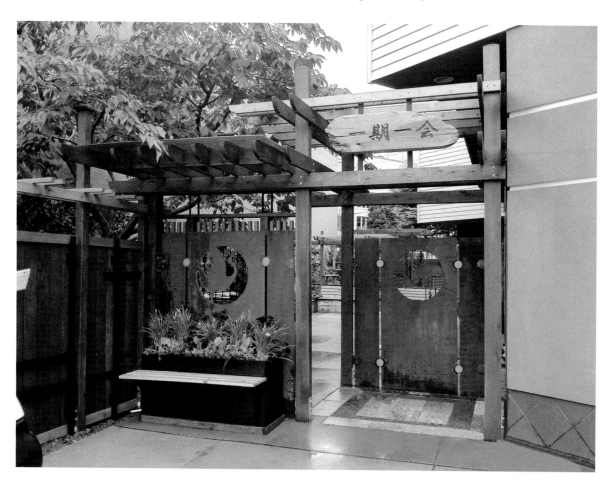

The crane motif integrated throughout the garden represents the cycle of life, good fortune, and longevity in Japanese culture and brings a sense of familiarity to the residents at Nikkei Manor.

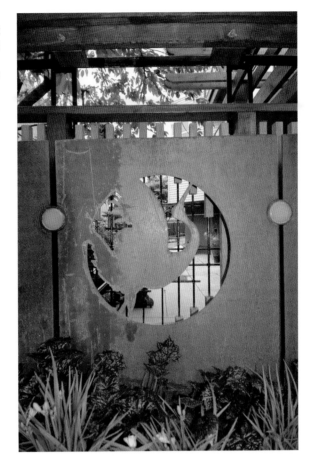

at the gate are a small crane with a fish and a larger crane with head tilted skyward; a third crane (elsewhere, near the emergency exit) is taking flight. In the process of designing the entry for cultural celebration and identity, one of the designers suggested naming the garden. The name chosen, *Ichi-go Ichi-e* ("one time, one meeting"), was carved in a wood sign and hung over the entry gate to be seen from the street.

To make the garden safe to use at night, a lighting plan was created. Uplights were used to illuminate the entry gate, water feature, cherry tree, Japanese maples, pavilion, Buddha, and emergency egress. Downlights were fitted along the ramps.

Grading

A major design concern is how to manage water as it travels through a garden, ideally in such a way that the shaping of the site offers therapeutic benefits. In most regions it is a sustainable benefit to keep rainwater on site to irrigate the planting areas, but when not controlled for water runoff, the garden's surfaces become puddled, eroded, muddy, mossy, or icy. However much the site naturally undulates, the designer is sculpting the ground plane to retain or create soft and hard surfaces, all needing drainage. Soft, planted earth forms include berms and swales or terraced beds. Hard surfaces include floors, paths, ramps, boardwalks, and decks, fabricated of concrete, stone, or wood. In directing surface water, one goal is to assure that the site will be universally accessible to garden users with mobility, balance, strength, dexterity, and sensory challenges. Examples show how, by artfully shaping and integrating the elevations of soft and hard surfaces, the designer can bring accessibility and usability, infuse the site with nature, and incorporate therapeutic benefits.

Universally accessible and engaging constructed and open spaces provide everyone with myriad places to play, learn, and move outdoors in all seasons.

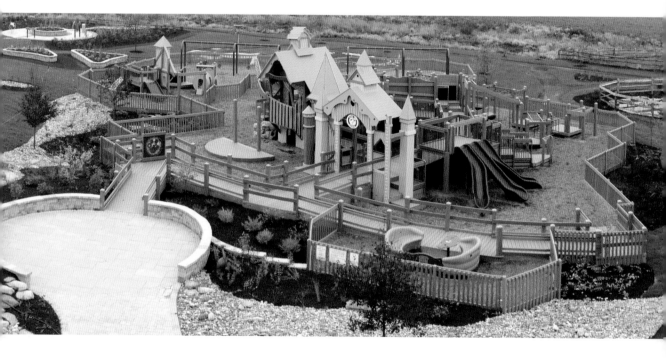

Slopes are calculated early in schematic design. On the flat areas of the site a minimum incline of one to two percent will drain water. When slopes are less than two percent, unit pavers will be difficult to lay with the required level of control; poured concrete or decomposed granite are alternatives. A slope is measured as rise over run. A line or path that rises to a height of one foot over a length or run of 50 feet is defined as 1:50 or expressed as a percent, $\frac{1}{50}$ equaling two percent. At two percent, a slope is just perceptible, and inclines of up to five percent are relatively easy for those using canes, walkers, and wheeled mobility devices to ascend or descend. Slopes greater than eight percent are not considered accessible. For slopes between five and eight percent, ADA code specifies how paths, ramps, landings, kick rails, and handrails should be detailed and dimensioned.

Introducing topographic change to a flat site can mitigate feelings of containment, claustrophobia, and boredom. Planted berms become points of focus that increase the depth of field and add a sense of mystery. Traditional Japanese gardens master this artful arrangement of grass, sand, or moss hills, where the visitor can visually or actually explore and

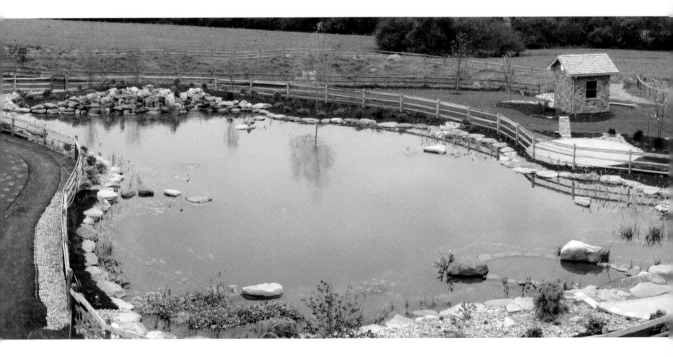

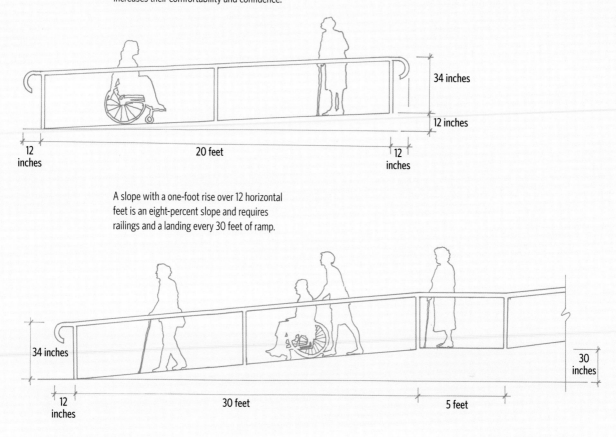

A slope with a one-foot rise over 20 horizontal feet is a five-percent slope and does not require railings, though for many users, having railings increases their comfortability and confidence.

34 inches

12 inches

12 inches

20 feet

12 inches

A slope with a one-foot rise over 12 horizontal feet is an eight-percent slope and requires railings and a landing every 30 feet of ramp.

34 inches

30 inches

12 inches

30 feet

5 feet

wander. At Incarnation Children's Center, a foster home in New York City for children with HIV/AIDS, a turf mound was created in a small courtyard garden as a soft surface for play. A broad and sloping wedge of earth and grass is enclosed on three sides by a timber frame structure rising to 30 inches. The sensory experience, as the children repeatedly climb and roll down their grassy hill, is absorbing and appealing.

When the site already has walled and retained elevations, the designer can take advantage of the height: placing a light canopy of small trees with an understory of flowering bulbs and perennials in a raised position softens the sense of enclosure. The plants, colors, textures, and scents have greater sensory impact if they are alongside integrated seating areas and walking paths. If the entire site is sloped, and the garden has different levels that need to be connected, ramps that are integrated into the design have therapeutic potential. Their gentle slopes can be used for exercise and rehabilitation. At five-percent grade or less, they readily accommodate, without too much challenge, walkers, wheelchairs, scooters, canes, strollers, and gurneys. A loop path linked by two ramps can be made more interesting if it ascends to and descends from an elevated landmark or destination. The destination might be some form of resting place, shelter, or viewpoint that provides a sense of being away.

The presence of hills on the site or near it create stimulating views to capture, especially if their colors, textures, and patterns are engaging. Mounds of aromatic lavender, or rowed fruit trees, or maples aflame with fall color offer sensory escape. At the Oklahoma City National Memorial, a field of empty chairs patterned up the slope of the hill expresses the stunning enormity and particularity of personal loss.

A design that captures rainwater at the site focuses on the essential, dynamic, and fascinating element of water. Designers cut a groove in the earth to make a swale that channels surface runoff to a raingarden that

Modest slopes can provide engaging play opportunities, even for children with serious illnesses, who will enjoy simply climbing up and rolling down the grassy incline.

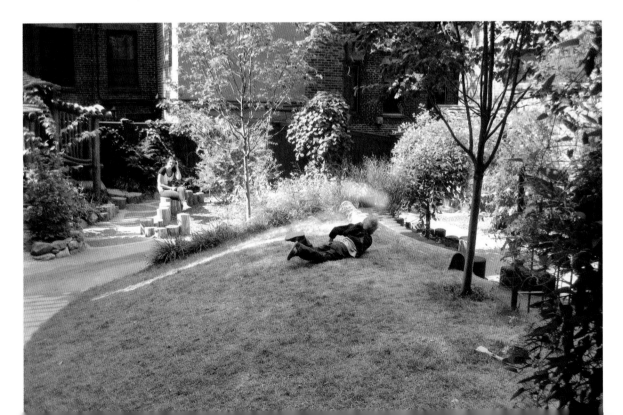

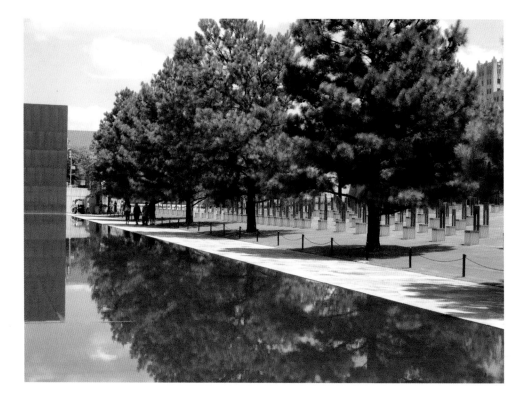

holds and infiltrates the water. Bioswales are planted with grasses, rushes, reeds, and sedges to filter pollutants, slowing the water and catching sediments to reduce erosion. The raingarden often has logs and snags for habitat enhancement and uses porous soils to percolate the water. Both systems are detailed and sized to be self-supporting and to deter standing water. Swales and raingardens bring birds, butterflies, and dragonflies into the garden.

Roof surfaces receive great amounts of rainwater. By directing it into an above or below ground cistern, the water is available when needed to irrigate the garden. In all these ways, garden users can witness natural systems at work in the garden. Water feeds the soils and plants, instead of heading to a wastewater treatment plant.

Empty chairs memorialize the 168 lives lost in the 1995 Oklahoma City bombing; the reflecting pool suggests the fluidity of life.

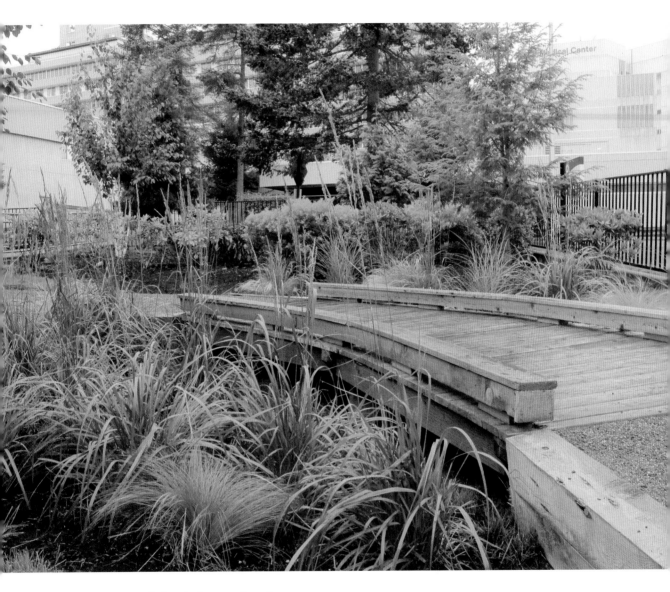

A raingarden is an appealing and
efficient way to avoid standing water
and feature a little-seen natural habitat.

Rooms

Designers commonly use the conceptual framework of rooms to organize and structure a garden. The carrying capacity of the entire site will dictate how many rooms of a determined size can be included. Rooms can be aligned along a passageway or corridor, radiate off a central space, or be linked room-to-room. A terminal room that has a single entry/exit can feel protected and private in a secure facility. Spaces can be arranged on a gradient from public to private, from noisy to quiet. This can be seen most simply in an arrangement of more quiet rooms off a central open space that is public, active, and noisy. The room opening, whether for entry or exit, establishes a threshold, a transition space that can be celebrated as such. The entries into the rooms can also be accentuated through scale, material, ornamentation, or color to emphasize the prominence of the space, to help direct users, or create a hierarchy between the various room options. For example, the primary entry from a building's interior into the garden can be a transitional space, allowing users to open an umbrella, adjust their eyes to the light, and identify landmarks and other features to draw them into the garden. Accentuating the threshold with an arbor modulates the experience of leaving or entering. In bright or sunny areas, screening overhead will make the transition between interior and natural light less jarring for older adults, those with autism spectrum disorder, and others who are photosensitive.

At the Tri-City Hospital in Oceanside, California, an at-grade courtyard garden is available to inpatients through sliding glass doors in their rooms; zero-step thresholds make for inclusive access. Another access, via electronically operated doors, is located close to the rehabilitation clinics; occupational, physical, and speech and language therapists can often be found in the courtyard with patients, working at umbrella-shaded tables, ambulating, or practicing other rehabilitation skills necessary for discharge. Besides being motivating, rehabilitation in an outdoor environment has the advantage of being realistic.

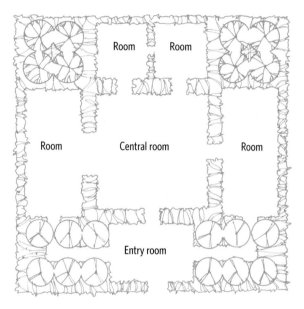

Room   Room

Room   Central room   Room

Entry room

Smaller rooms can be organized around a central primary space, used for gathering and large activities, that feeds into them.

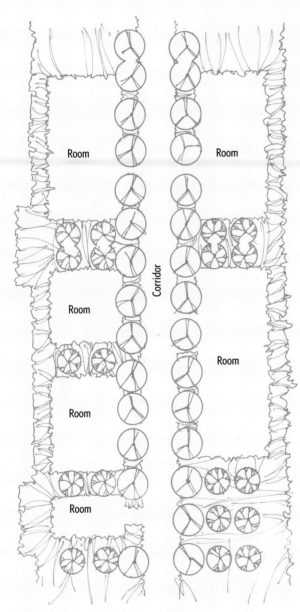

Rooms can also be organized along a corridor, a strategy often used in tight lineal spaces.

Room

Room

Corridor

Room

Room

Room

Room

Room

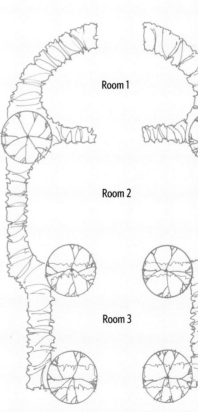

Rooms can be linked; however, this circulation pattern can impinge on a user's need for privacy. Often a variety of strategies are used within a garden.

Room 1

Room 2

Room 3

Oregon Burn Center

The Oregon Burn Center Garden at Legacy Emanuel Medical Center in Portland, Oregon, is the first therapeutic garden in the United States designed for those who have survived burns. Using a room-to-room organizational structure, designer Brian Bainnson of Quatrefoil, Inc., created a series of flowing spaces. To achieve visual separation, many of the spaces are surrounded with dense plantings, architectural screens, and trees, and the circular arrangement of several spaces allows users to skirt occupied spaces, respecting each other's privacy. The garden is enclosed by patient rooms on two sides and a steel fence and dense plantings on the other two. Access to it is restricted to staff, families, and patients, many of whom are significantly disfigured by their traumatic injury. This intentionally private courtyard garden is used for rehabilitation, visiting, and escape; it is a place where those learning to accept their physical transformation feel safe and protected. Patients, accompanied by staff or family, are guided through the garden rooms, stopping to touch ornamental flowers, smell herbs, or harvest fruit and vegetables.

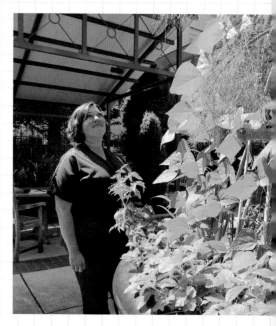

One enters the space via a gently downsloping ramp. The eye focuses on a solitary basalt column, with water flowing down its rough surface—a landmark that signals entry into a multisensory space where patients begin the arduous journey of physical and emotional rehabilitation. The first room is circular, with a raised planter in its center and several benches where patients can rest and regain stamina beneath the dappled shade of birches and vine maples. This room abuts the second and largest room, which features a circular lawn surrounded by a pathway. On one side, an intimate room-within-a-room is marked by four columns supporting a vine-covered roof plane; there, patients and family sit and converse while watching their children, many of whom are patients at play. A red miniature firehouse is filled with child-sized riding toys; a "retired" firefighter waterhose hangs on its side. This whimsical play element is also an important therapy element requested by the therapy team: uncoiling and rolling it up requires strength, balance, coordination, and endurance. A red hydrant,

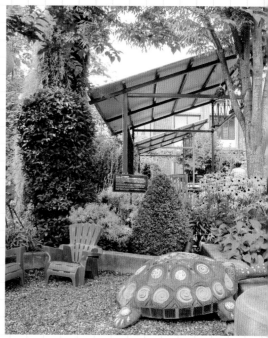

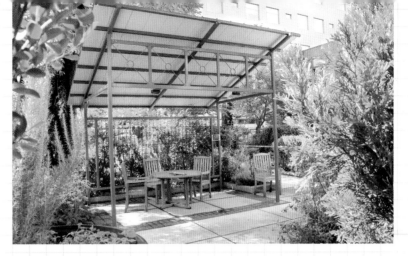

RIGHT Pavilions provide shade—or cover from the Oregon rain. Tables and chairs allow patients and staff to engage in activities they would typically do indoors.

OPPOSITE TOP Staff find respite in the garden's quiet spaces and abundant, often edible plantings. This container overflows with tomatoes, strawberries, fennel, and sweet potato vine.

OPPOSITE BOTTOM The scale of many garden elements is specifically sized for children and allows for intergenerational participation.

used for watering plants and play, may seem incongruous at a burn center, but the design was discussed with staff therapists and approved. Firefighters help save lives, and they are one reason the patients, despite their ordeal, are alive—a hopeful counterpoint to the pain of their trauma.

Next, a tiny room is set with brightly colored child-sized chairs and tiled turtle statues, ready for children to sit in or scramble over, respectively. Just beyond, another small room with movable furniture offers staff respite from their intensive jobs and is designated for their use only. The final room is a long, narrow space, featuring two covered steel pavilions with wooden tables and seating arranged for meetings, eating, writing, and physical and occupational therapy intervention. Surrounding these structures are colorful pots tucked between dense plantings of edible and sensory perennials and intermixed with evergreen shrubs; these last provide year-round presence, color, and separation between the garden rooms. There are ample characterful spaces to walk and wheel on varied surfaces within this courtyard garden; and paths flanked with steel railings are often used for physical rehabilitation.

Railings support physical rehabilitation. Rooms are screened with vegetation, encouraging exploration while providing sanctuaries of solitude and transition for patients with serious burn injuries.

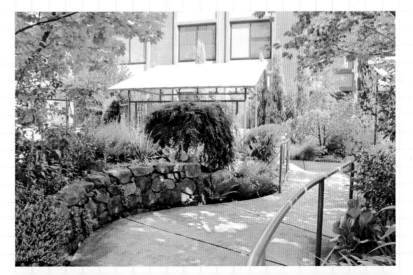

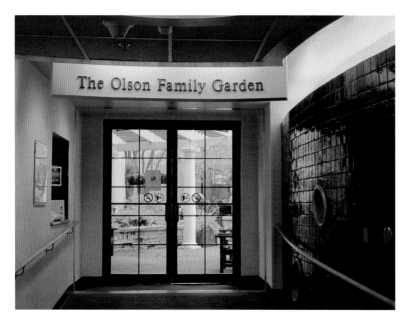

Transitions between interior and exterior spaces enable users to pause until their eyes adjust to the change in light.

Spaces can be separated in various subtle ways. Spaces separated by a lattice screen wall create semi-privacy and allow for different activities in each space while maintaining some connection; this might be important to promote safety or prevent feelings of isolation. Two spaces lacking vertical wall definition, with just a slight change of paving material or an elevation of the ground plane, can support activities that overlap, as for instance providing a social gathering space for parents that abuts a play area for young children, or, as at Nikkei Manor, the spaces that functioned together as performance stage and audience seating.

STRUCTURING SPATIAL VOLUME

A room is constructed of planes: the walls or vertical planes, the floor or ground plane, and the ceiling or overhead plane. These elements are the designer's tools for spatial and aesthetic differentiation. The proportions and materials of these planes elicit a range of reactions and feelings among users. The presence or absence of these elements will bring out different responses. A solid, overhead plane reinforces a sense of enclosure, and its absence evokes feelings of openness and expansion. When built like an arbor (that is, with structural elements widely spaced), the overhead plane has a degree of translucency and openness. Adding a thick covering of vines, it becomes more opaque, like a solid ceiling. Many aspects of materiality come into play—color, texture, tactility, movement. A brick wall conveys a formality absent in a bamboo hedge that sways

A room consists of three planes: 1. the walls or vertical planes, 2. the floor or ground plane, and 3. the ceiling or roof plane.

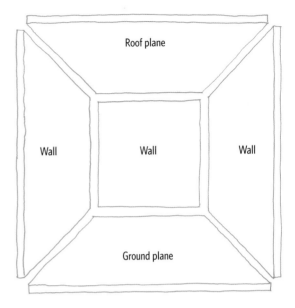

Roof plane

Wall

Wall

Wall

Ground plane

The flowing form of Bronson Methodist Hospital's atrium garden is balanced with small nooks created by plantings for quiet meditation and reflection.

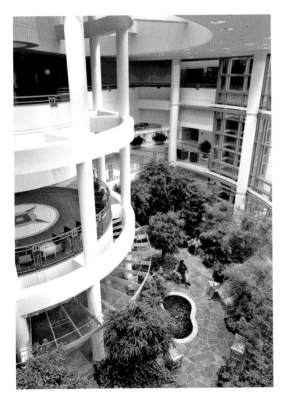

and rustles with the wind and, though visually dense, feels less solid. A clipped evergreen hedge and a stone wall will be experienced as two very different expressions of "border."

ROOM SIZE AND SHAPE

The size and shape of the room—circular, rectilinear, or free-form—will evoke different feelings and suggest different activities. Some shapes, circles for example, are archetypal and can be used to accentuate focusing, mystery, and connectivity. Larger, more free-form organic shapes might foster wandering, exploration, and discovery. Small spaces in a therapeutic garden have enclosure, privacy, and safety, which are compatible for meditation, intimate conversation, and grieving. A garden for people with dementia is most beneficial if it is small and contained, with open sightlines, simple spatial divisions, and clear wayfinding; the advantages are that patients will not get lost or confused, which can quickly elevate their anxiety level and lead to agitation.

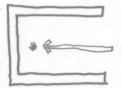

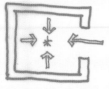

Available space is only one consideration when deciding upon the shape of a room. The decision is also based on what users and activities the room will support, what feelings it should evoke, and how it fits within the garden composition.

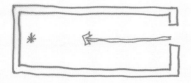

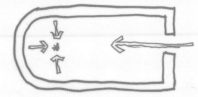

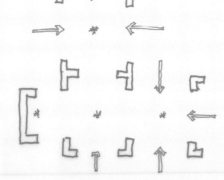

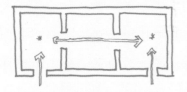

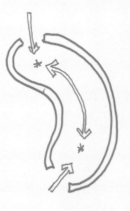

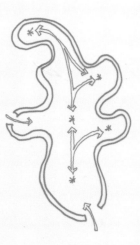

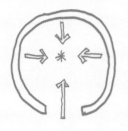

FLEXIBLE SPACES

Multiple-function spaces build flexibility into the design, allowing activities to be either concurrently or consecutively scheduled. For example, a small rectangular space will function like a living or family room; if the furniture is not built in, chairs and tables and wheeled devices can be arranged for the greatest variety of activities and numbers of people. Devices for various therapies—adjustable-height tables, roll-down flooring, planting and water-play carts—can be brought in as needed. Movable partitions, privacy shades, and planters on rollers are useful to transform a large space into two smaller ones. Sound is difficult to block with such temporary divisions but can be buffered by vertical vegetation and masked by a burbling water feature. Less prescriptive design that offers flexible configurations will support programs that may change in the future. With this flexibility, a room could be a place for a staff yoga class before work, one-on-one speech therapy in the morning, physical rehabilitation after lunch, an eating disorder support group in the afternoon, and casual socializing in the evening.

Cancer Lifeline in Seattle is a resource for those diagnosed with cancer

A view through the wood doors, from Sky toward Earth. Ornamental grasses, fuchsias, geraniums, and other perennials enclose the space, and all seating has armrests, as nausea and balance problems associated with motion upon rising often trouble people with cancer.

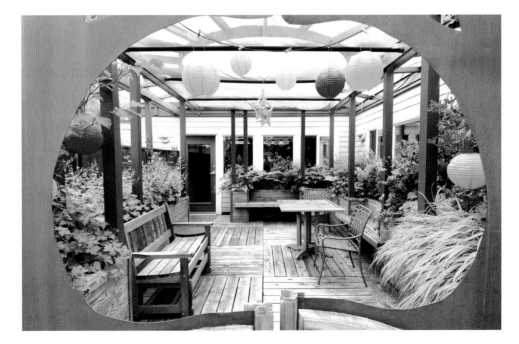

and their family members. A series of therapeutic gardens was created in three locations on the second-story rooftop of their center. The largest of these, the Earth and Sky garden, occupies an L-shaped space designed for multiple functions. The Earth garden abuts an interior room for art therapy classes, which can readily spill out into the garden. The room is surrounded with planters for therapeutic horticultural activities; when furniture is brought in, the space is used by clients and their families for counseling and support groups. The Sky garden is an open and casual social space with movable furniture and a two-seat glider oriented to views of the neighborhood and the Cascade Mountains. Wood doors separating the two spaces are inlaid with hammered copper sheets with cutouts portraying the tree of life, a powerful healing element for mature patients. The doors also operate as a curtain for a puppet stage (counselors use puppets and other pretend play methods with children as a means of talking about the emotional issues surrounding cancer). The two spaces, Earth and Sky, flow as one for gatherings and memorials. Two other gardens—a kitchen garden and a garden for grief and meditation—are separately accessed.

MULTIPLE ROOMS

The advantage of a large garden with multiple rooms is that it offers choices, which can relieve anxiety for those whose sense of control is diminished by their loss of well-being. Having compassionately understood users through participatory design, the designer orchestrates these choices into a sequence of rooms. How these rooms are sized, shaped, and refined will affect not just what people do in the garden but how it feels to be there. The experiences of familiarity and belonging, mystery and wonder reduce stress, especially when people are confined and controlled, confused, or disconnected by their environment or routines.

The gardens at Canuck House in Vancouver, B.C., offer a grounding sense of home to children in hospice care and their families. The garden rooms are sequenced off a loop path beginning at the side door of the estate house. The backyard tone is set at the garden's threshold by an enclosure of trees and understory plants with birdhouses, birdbaths, and natural stone water fountains. Next is a covered open-sided pavilion with a fireplace wall and hearth, dining table, and cooking grill.

OPPOSITE LEFT Being offered the opportunity to gather flowers from a cutting garden and bring them inside to a loved one's room can positively influence sense of control and meaning for family members.

OPPOSITE RIGHT This garden room, one of a series of "crying rooms," provides comfort with familiar elements and creates privacy with stone walls and a recirculating wall fountain, which muffles the sounds of pain and grief.

In hospice gardens, families, especially those with children, need to have a safe and accessible outlet for play, even when dealing with end-of-life issues.

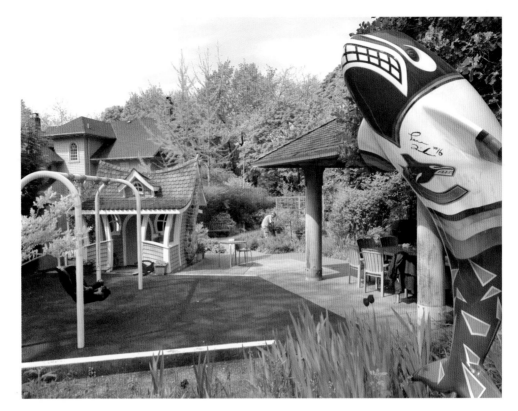

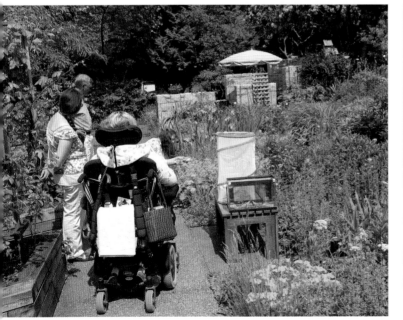

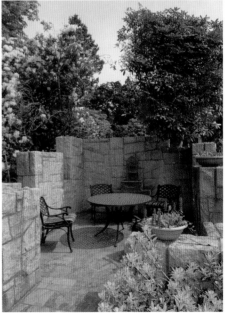

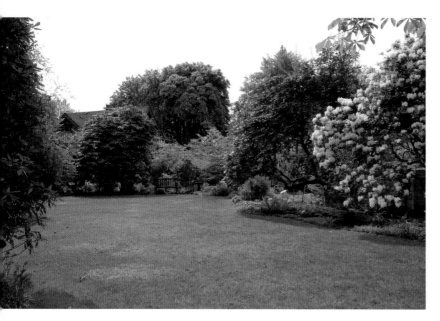

Open, soft green rooms full of near and far nature inspire movement and offer fascination and sensory experiences.

Contiguous to the family gathering area is a children's imaginative play space, centered on an eccentric playhouse, all curvilinear, at once novel and straight from a picture book. Children can take a ramp to an upper play area with a merry-go-round that spins flush to the ground. A recurring theme of flowers on the low concrete partition walls is rendered in painted murals. By these continuous measures of familiarity and wonder, children and their parents find both belonging and escape, and some relief from the anxiety associated with terminal illness and dislocation from home.

The children pass next through an herb garden to arrive at a production garden and cutting garden—a great attraction for butterflies and the children themselves, who like to carry the flowers back to their rooms. The edible garden has raised beds and trellises for growing berries, peas, and beans, which children harvest and take to the kitchen for cooking. Nearby is a small grieving room, a simple stone enclosure with plants and seating and water feature. When children follow a serpentine path, they discover a large open lawn surrounded by trees; in this large green room, the children are completely immersed in nature, choosing either the wonder of grass and open sky or the fascination of exploring the layers of shrubs, trees, and hiding places at its crenelated edges. These experiences reduce stress and, for the families, reinvigorate memories of home, before the onset of illness.

A ROOM WITH A VIEW

Some gardens are designed simply for viewing. Evidence shows that the therapeutic experience of nature is a benefit to all, even those who need to remain inside for their care or treatment. For example, Nakamura and Fujii (1990) compared the outcomes of patients with a view of even a simple potted plant versus those with only a view of a human-made object or a pot without the plant. Brain wave activity was monitored, and those viewing the plant were found to be more wakefully relaxed.

The most effective location for a viewing garden is contiguous to a common gathering area with a full window wall. The designer orients the plants and other natural features to the windows. Flowering specimen trees, ornamental grasses, conifers, and broadleaf evergreens can provide fascination and beauty in every season. The seating in the interior rooms will need to be arranged to allow unobstructed access to garden views by both ambulatory and wheeled mobility users.

The garden can also be brought into the building; greenhouses, warm, fragrant, and full of light, offer great possibilities for use during cold winter months when the outdoor garden may be less interesting or inviting. For those confined to a hospital room, on bed rest, and on strict infection-control precautions, a view of even a small garden can reduce stress and offers both a sense of escape and a reconnection to the dynamic natural world outside.

A view of nature from inside a rehabilitation clinic may be as motivating as being outdoors for patients receiving occupational and physical therapy.

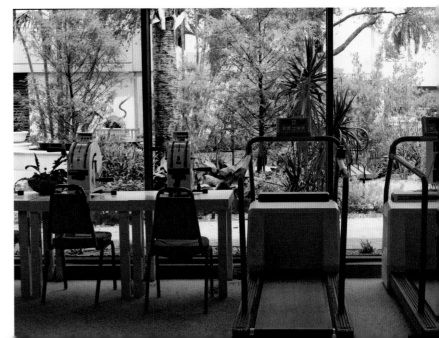

The Stoneman Healing Garden at the Dana-Farber Cancer Institute in Boston offers quiet respite, exotic escape, and meets the stringent standards for infection control: patients unable to be outdoors can enter a self-contained plexiglass area with unobstructed views of the garden, which is planted with bamboos, ornamental gingers, orchids, and other tropical plants. Semi-private, flexible and fixed seating options enable users to find a comfortable place to appreciate the plantings or take in the city through floor-to-ceiling windows. The curves and angles of the garden create options for how and where to be in the garden, and lighting encourages use during the day and evening.

Whether viewed from within or without, the garden maintains its therapeutic sensory appeal through a thoughtful balance of color, height, texture, plants, and other natural elements such as river rocks and wood.

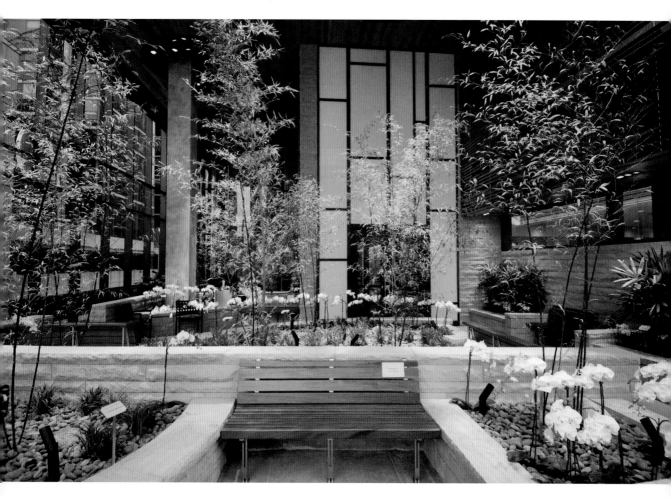

Paths

Paths provide many therapeutic benefits in the garden. They offer connection to nature, the chance for private conversation, fresh-air exercise, and meditative walking. Paths that provide a sense of mystery and escape need a proportional dose of clarity and coherence. If a path's direction, pattern, and flow are too unpredictable, certain users—those with dementia, post-traumatic stress disorder (PTSD), or autism spectrum disorder, for example—will avoid entering. At the same time, a path comprehended entirely at the outset lacks allure and interest. A person struggling with uncertainty in the trajectory of their illness will be more sensitive to incoherence in their environment. The designer respects these user needs by finding the right balance of mystery and clarity in the composition of the paths.

Functional paths (connecting, say, a parking lot with a point of entry) are usually direct and efficient. As soon as a path bends, it invites the traveler to slow down and take in the surroundings. Winding paths in a garden may offer the deepest experiences of therapeutic relief and

This universally designed path balances mystery with clarity. The curves add a sense of anticipation, but because the plantings are low enough, users are able to see what lies ahead.

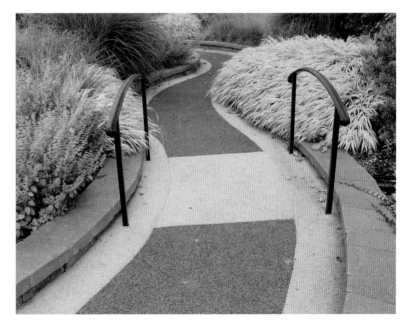

respite; moving forward, immersed in verdant plantings, whether alone or with a companion, the traveler has a chance to reflect and wonder. As the landscape unfolds, the new and familiar intersect. The person in motion is anchored by the comfort and connection of familiar landmarks like a specimen tree or boulder, even as his or her senses are stirred to take in changing sounds, sights, textures, and scents. Variability engages interest and lets the mind escape from stressful and intrusive thoughts and anxious feelings. A single serpentine path with slight elevation changes will bring users out into the garden. Wandering beneath a canopy of trees, users can experience the shifting quality of light and air. Loop paths of various lengths allow users to find one that corresponds to their capabilities and endurance.

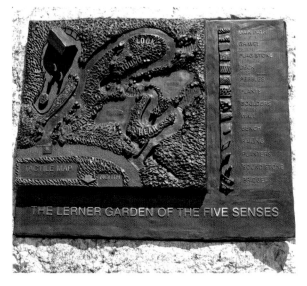

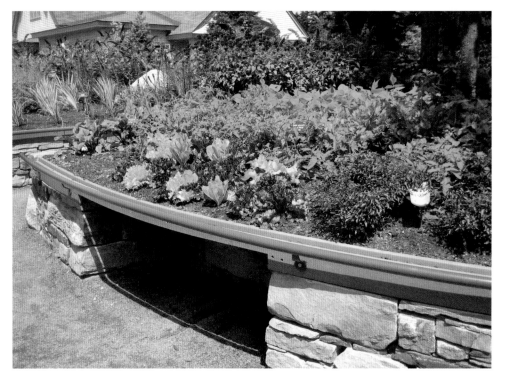

TOP A tactile relief map welcomes those with visual challenges.

BOTTOM Cutouts in the raised tasting beds allow wheeled mobility users to roll under the beds and explore the plantings. An integrated handrail system running along the perimeter enables people to safely navigate the space.

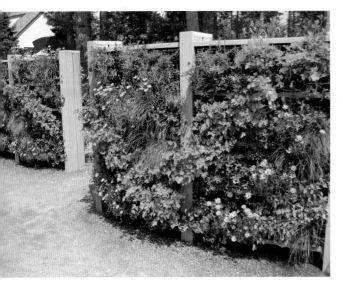

Vertical gardens planted in a rippling wave pattern are inviting for seated and standing visitors to see and touch.

The Lerner Garden of the Five Senses is an interactive sensory garden designed as a single looping and meandering path with a separate entry and exit off a main pathway. Located near the visitor center at the Coastal Maine Botanical Gardens, the garden is meant to sharpen a guest's senses as a prelude to exploring the rest of the 250-acre waterfront garden. Landscape architect Herb Schaal worked with people who are blind to understand how to incorporate sensory cues for wayfinding and accessibility. At the arched entry, a granite boulder presents the visitor with a tactile garden map on a cast bronze plaque. The path's winding descent leads to a bridge that separates the upper and lower ponds and then ascends to an exit. The path orchestrates a coherent and sequenced series of experiences of natural phenomena, beginning with the sense of smell. The ground plane of the scent nook has a perceptible tactile change of pattern in the stone, signaling there is a turnout in the path, and the path itself has a continuous striker-stone at one raised edge, which serves people using white canes for orientation and mobility.

The path is wide enough for two wheelchairs to travel side by side, and the grades are less than five percent. At every point along the path, the sound of water from the heart of the garden's center is heard. The largest nook is the tasting garden, where waist-high beds offer choices of edible fruits, flowers, leaves, and seeds in a variety of sweet, savory, minty, and bitter flavors. Raised planter beds for wheelchair users to roll under are designed to meet the ADA code at 27 inches of clearance; scooter users need 30 inches. Both heights are also appropriate for standing gardeners.

The plants in the "look" nook present a visual smorgasbord of color, shape, and size. From its higher elevation, views are framed inward to the ponds and outward to the layered landscape of the rest of the botanic garden. In this way, the grade change brings spatial depth and a sense of visual escape. The next nook near the ponds features a reflexology labyrinth and many textural plants to touch. The fifth zone, the sound nook, has hollowed stone sculptures that act like musical instruments; by humming or talking into the holes, visitors hear sounds resonate. A second bridge, crossing a creek burbling out from the upper pond, signals the garden's exit.

CLOSER LOOK

VA Puget Sound Fisher House

The therapeutic garden at the VA Puget Sound Fisher House was completed by two University of Washington landscape architecture design/build studios, both directed by Daniel Winterbottom. Fisher House provides a welcoming home for military families whose loved one is receiving long- or short-term treatment at a VA hospital; the intent of the therapeutic garden at the Fisher House was to extend that sense of home and to restore and inspire all who enter it. The project began with the transformation of an existing suburban landscape into a therapeutic garden, dedicated in June 2010; the final phase of the garden was completed and dedicated in June 2013.

The participatory design process included multiple face-to-face meetings with a panel of house guests, Fisher House and VA staff, University of Washington landscape architecture faculty and local landscape architects, and Seattle garden club members to explain and showcase the various design options put forth by the design/build studio students. The panel also took part in surveys and photo-preference boards to further inform the design process. The therapeutic garden, which now encompasses the entirety of the outdoor space at the house, is an oasis for families and Fisher House staff. Universal design elements include a wide, smooth loop path (a 0.12 mile circuit) that easily accommodates a pair of wheeled mobility devices traveling in tandem. A stage, accessible to all by a gently sloped ramp or stairs, hosts yoga and other activities. A kick railing increases the safety and usability of the bridge spanning the raingarden. Multiple raised planters filled with herbs and vegetables, including one with a cantilevered edge, enable users of all ages and abilities to tend produce destined for the kitchen.

One way to enter the space is through a kitchen garden, leading to a central plaza. The focal point

LEFT In and out of the shelter, screening behind the seating comforts veterans with PTSD, who need protected, defensible spaces to feel at ease. Space between the benches accommodates wheeled mobility users as equals and allows those who prefer to stand to do so.

RIGHT This calming water feature provides audio and visual sensorial engagements. The rock—split apart but rejoined by healing water—is a metaphor for veterans and their families.

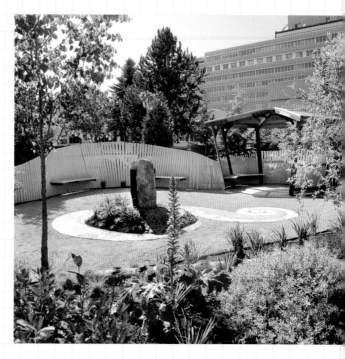

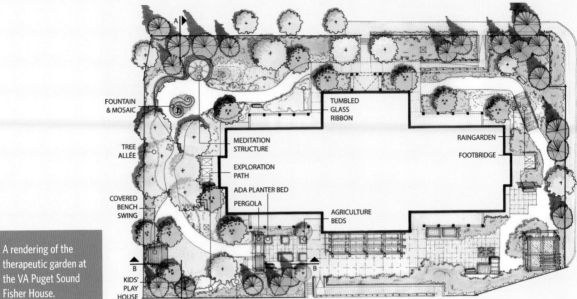

FOUNTAIN & MOSAIC

TREE ALLÉE

COVERED BENCH SWING

KIDS' PLAY HOUSE

MEDITATION STRUCTURE

EXPLORATION PATH

ADA PLANTER BED

PERGOLA

TUMBLED GLASS RIBBON

AGRICULTURE BEDS

RAINGARDEN

FOOTBRIDGE

WILLOW PLAY STRUCTURE

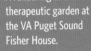

A rendering of the therapeutic garden at the VA Puget Sound Fisher House.

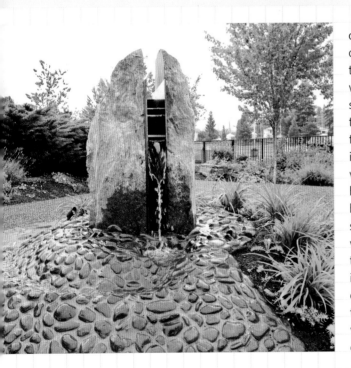

of the plaza is a "reflection" sculpture composed of copper bands weaving through a bed of ornamental grasses, suggesting the movement of wind and water. Aromatic plants, rocks, and logs nourish the senses with texture and color. A raingarden, adjacent to another plaza, captures water on site. A meditation shelter, sited to offer views of Mount Rainier, welcomes all users to come inside. An extended woodland restoration garden with an at-grade bridge completes the "healing journey," symbolizing both spiritual and ecological reclamation. There are spaces for children to play, for people to sit alone or with others, to engage in gentle exercise, to nourish the senses, and to garden. Those who spend time in the garden—socializing, reflecting, walking—feel enriched and restored. Because of the many choices the garden provides, users are able to do what they want and need to do in a safe and enveloping outdoor environment.

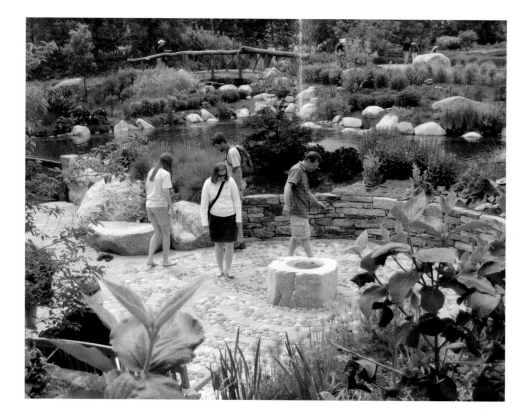

Labyrinths or mazes have long been a feature of garden design. More complex designs, with meandering multiple courses, are meant to be puzzles to solve; some paths lead to dead ends so the visitor is typically lost or briefly confused before finding the exit or the goal of the center point. In the extravagant palace and estate gardens of 17th-century France, hedge mazes in the gardens were a pleasant diversion that relieved the monotony of walks. In therapeutic gardens, where the intent is to give the user opportunities to restore mental focus, to meditate, or to perform a spiritual ritual, a labyrinth need not be challenging. When a labyrinth is intended to be meditative, it is best to locate it in a more remote section of the therapeutic garden. If designed for walking, the path can be made narrow and will achieve some length; the labyrinth at Chartres cathedral, for example, has a path 450 feet long.

A unicursal labyrinth is one continuous path on a two-dimensional plane. The simplest form is a compact spiral ending in a center point, as in the touch zone at the Lerner Garden, where the circular form of a labyrinth is rendered as a reflexology path, made of smooth local river stones of graduated sizes (reflexology, an ancient healing art common in Asia, is

The path leads to a river rock labyrinth, best experienced with bare feet. Lush plantings and local glacial rocks add to the garden's sensory appeal.

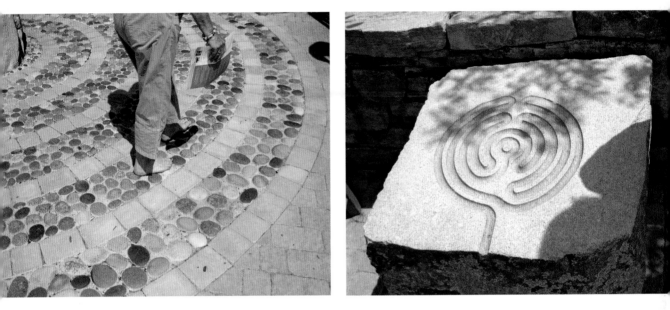

LEFT Polished river rocks integrated into a reflexology path add to the tactile experience.

RIGHT Those unable to navigate the reflexology path can use their hands or fingers to trace a replica of the labyrinth, carved into a nearby flat stone.

the stimulation of acupressure points to improve circulation and reduce overall stress). The 12-inch-wide river rock path at Lerner is meant to be walked in bare feet; it is edged by cobblestones and makes multiple turns leading to the center. Arriving there, visitors touch a soft layer of moss in a depression atop a granite boulder—a sensation that contrasts with the hard river rocks below.

PATH-DESIGN DETAILS

The detailing of paths and surfaces will determine the garden's universal accessibility, how easily it will accommodate the widest range of users. A six- to eight-foot-wide path allows two people in wheelchairs to pass or stroll together easily; similarly, wheeled mobility users, scooters, powered wheelchairs, and gurneys can move in tandem with a person using no mobility devices or with a parent pushing a carriage. Primary paths need to be wide enough to accommodate sociable interaction; a seven- to eight-foot-wide path might be considered. For secondary and solitary pathways, or where space is very limited, the path should not be less than three feet wide to accommodate all types of mobility. The path will need to provide frequent rest spots for those who are ill, in pain, or who move with great effort, needing breaks. Depending on user needs,

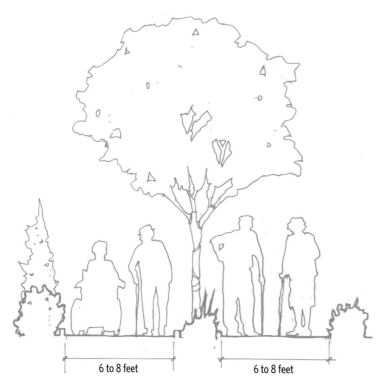

6 to 8 feet   6 to 8 feet

A path width of six to eight feet will accommodate two people or two wheelchairs side by side.

seating options or turnout areas should be placed frequently along the walking path.

MATERIALS SELECTION

The selection of surface and supporting materials will impact who can use the path and how easy and comfortable the experience will be. Some materials should probably be avoided as they tend to be slippery, difficult to walk on, or see. Mulch lacks the firmness and traction needed by users with canes, crutches, walkers, or wheels. Crushed gravel or shell meets ADA standards and is economical, but this surface can be a challenge for wheeled mobility users to navigate and for people with balance issues. Those sensitive to touch and sound may find the crunching feel underfoot and the sound distressing as well.

Brick, smooth cut stone, slate, and river rocks pose problems when used in wet climates and where moss is prevalent. With a minimal amount of moisture, all become very difficult to navigate and anyone with balance or mobility problems will find them uncomfortable. Pea gravel or round small stones that move under foot also cause balance problems and tripping hazards; they should not be used.

The most accommodating surface is asphalt or cast-in-place concrete, tinted, brushed, or mixed with aggregate to reduce glare. The concrete should be crack-free, with joint spaces no greater than ⅛ inch. This assures that walker, crutch, or cane tips, IV poles, or shoe heels will not get stuck and cause a fall. Precast concrete pavers or textured stone pavers can also provide a consistent, durable, and aesthetic type of paving. When dry laid, care needs to be taken to ensure the joints are very tight and that there is no settlement of the base courses that will result in an uneven wearing course. The pavers can also be mortar-set on a concrete slab or raised on a pedestal system in roof gardens. They are available in various colors, textures, and shapes.

It is good practice to avoid light colors for paving, as the reflective surfaces of white marble, very light concrete, or gravel can temporarily blind users. High-contrast pattern in paving can be disorienting for people with low vision, autism, dementia, or some psychological issues. In high-contrast paving patterns, dark segments may be perceived not as paving

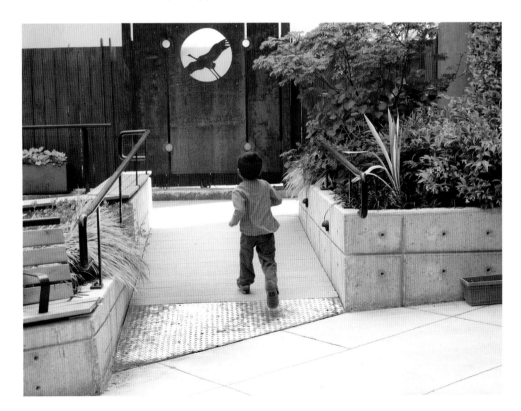

A visual and tactile metal warning strip informs users of a change in grade.

but rather as holes, so the path will be avoided. It is better to express pattern with subtle differentiations of color, tones, and texture. Warning strips to alert users of grade changes, at the beginning of a slope or stairs, for example, are also helpful, especially for users who are visually impaired.

Paths should be edged with curbs six inches high or greater to ensure that people and wheels stay on the path. The visual cue is accented when the edge color or material contrasts with the path appearance, offering a guide for those with low vision and those using canes or other walking supports. Curved edging can be made of steel, aluminum, or concrete, segmented courses of wood, stone, or brick units.

Boardwalks are often used for the same purpose as paths. Boardwalks that become bridges crossing over vegetation or water can be an intriguing change of experience. When boardwalks or bridges are used, kick rails are necessary to prevent those with diminished sight or perceptual issues (such as are caused by multiple sclerosis) and users with walkers, canes, crutches, or wheeled mobility devices from going over the edge. Kick rails are usually made of wood or metal and should be six to eight inches high to prevent tripping.

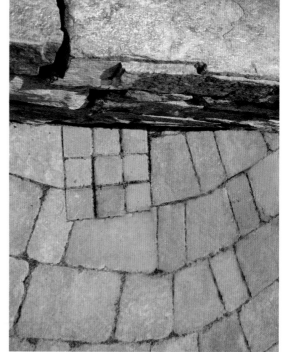

The nine small square pavers indicate a directional change is ahead for people with blindness or low vision who use white canes.

The ramp is a wonderful playful element of design, not just an accessible path or stair alternative. Ramps can easily take on a serpentine form, winding through vegetation and descending into the garden in a graceful sweep. When well designed, they can be used by physical and occupational therapists for rehabilitation, and all their clients will be readily accommodated. Ramps do consume more room than stairs, so maximizing their benefits as therapy program elements will help justify their place in a design when space is short.

ADA guidelines require 42-inch-high guardrails for ramps, landings, or stairs that are higher than 30 inches from finish grade. Also, handrails 34 to 38 inches in height are required for all ramps with an incline of eight percent; integrating handrails on boardwalks, bridges, and gentle ramps gives users confidence in their own safety and support. Local building code should be reviewed prior to design or replacement. Guardrails and

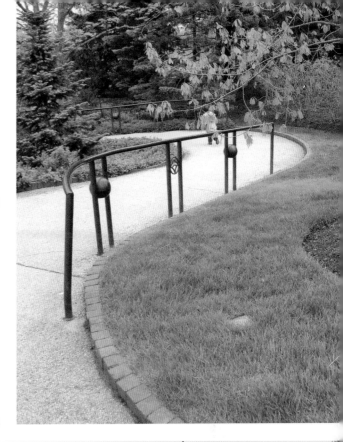

TOP Where does the path end and the garden bed begin? Even low edging provides both a visual and tactile cue.

BOTTOM Kick rails are another important safety and sensory feature; they too ensure that wheels and feet stay on track.

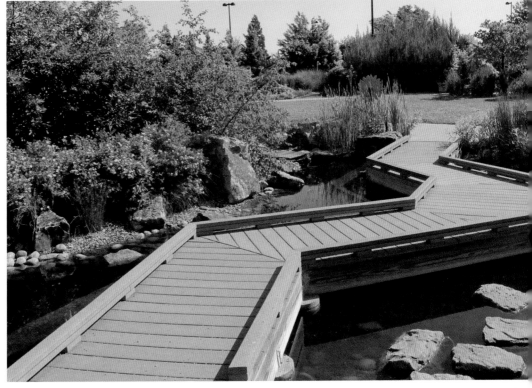

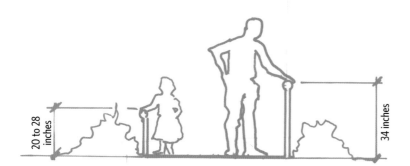

20 to 28 inches

34 inches

For many users, railings along paths provide critical support and wayfinding. They should be sized for the intended users.

handrails along steps, ramps, and paths need not be purely utilitarian; blended with the landscape they can simultaneously comply with ADA standards and be attractive. A slightly textured surface will keep hands from slipping off the railings. Multiple level rails oriented in parallel enable users of different heights to access the railings easily.

Integrating parallel bars along a path offers users opportunities to practice ambulation and balance skills. The majority of parallel bars for indoor use are adjustable in height from 26 to 44 inches; when parallel bars are incorporated as a fixed part of the frame design of a garden structure, one at 29 inches and one at 38 inches will accommodate a wider range of users.

Plants

With all the hardscape (including arbors, planters, paths, and seating) complete, the plants often enter all at once near the end of a therapeutic garden installation. A frenzy of placement—of specimen trees, mounding shrubs and perennials, carpeting groundcovers—instantly brings the project to life. But from the earliest phases of design, the designer has thought about the plants, how they will shape the spaces of the garden through the four seasons and successfully thrive on the site over time. The plants are the spiritual essence of the garden. They tell the story of emergence, growth, maturation, transformation, and renewal. The designer narrates this story by choosing plants whose multisensory qualities relate to the users.

Responses to color vary among users, in association with both individual and cultural preferences. Some users might favor the vivid boldness

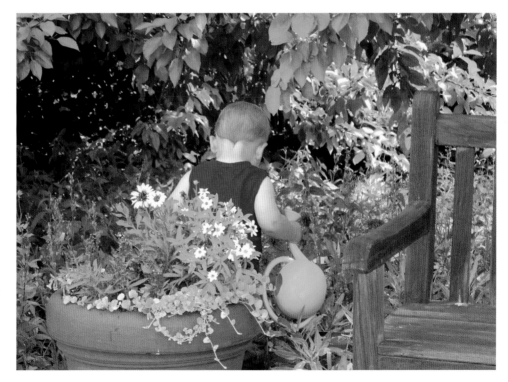

Being in a garden rich with multisensory elements is an immersive, nurturing experience for all ages.

of bright annuals and perennials; others, especially those in a state of heightened anxiety and stress, may prefer the subtlety of nuanced colors. Meditative gardens call for a quiet composition of plants—fine-leafed vines like akebia, softly blanketing mosses, rustling bamboo. Users with certain psychological conditions such as PTSD or anxiety disorder may be overstimulated by too much visual contrast and activity in the garden and will find comfort in a more minimalistic meditative retreat.

Highly aromatic herbs are welcome additions to sensory gardens and therapeutic programming at behavioral health and memory care facilities. Beyond the immediate sensory experience, users benefit if plants trigger a sense of wonder because they are unfamiliar or, conversely, a sense of belonging or connection because they are familiar. The Garden of Fragrance in the San Francisco Botanical Garden, designed in 1965 for visitors with visual impairments, has a loop path with 12 stations at beds raised to place a profusion of herbs within reach of wheelchair users. Visitors touch the cascading branches of rosemary leaves on a rock wall, release its scent, and may think of home cooking.

Plants that trigger positive memories of home because of their sweet or savory or unusual scents are especially meaningful to people displaced because of illness, homelessness, or unfamiliar relocation. The evocative scents of sage or rose can engender a comfortable sense of belonging to people in elder care facilities. Used as a tea, the smell and very fine texture of chamomile is universally well loved; the fragrance of both it and lavender are found to improve mood and ease stress. People may find the smell of lemon, mint, or strongly aromatic marigolds either invigorating or overwhelming. Children with sensory and movement disorders may be particularly sensitive to aversive textures, so soft turf grasses need to be selected for them. For children with sensory challenges, learning to touch, smell, and talk about the plants may be one goal in their structured occupational or speech therapy programs.

Herbs that have medicinal properties are often used in therapeutic gardens. For the garden she designed at Marin General Hospital's Cancer Center, Topher Delaney chose, among others with similar significance, Madagascar periwinkle (*Catharanthus roseus*), which contains alkaloids used to create the cancer drugs vinblastine and vincristine. Though the active ingredients used in most cancer treatments are now synthetic, it is meaningful to the patients who contemplate them that the plants in their therapeutic garden were the original and natural source of their healing drugs.

NATURAL CYCLES

There are plants that throughout the day and the seasons celebrate vitality and transformation within their natural context. In the garden, this can connect users to their place in the natural cycle. Plants like miscanthus, placed to catch early morning or evening light, mark the opening and passing of the day. In a bed of red and white flowers viewed day and night, the red ones pop at noon and disappear at night, when the whites take the stage, turning luminous. In four-season climates, the garden can be designed to unfold in a sequence of emergence, bloom, and return to the earth. Early bulbs and other spring ephemerals erupt as daylight lengthens, before the deciduous trees leaf out, followed by perennials. As the days shorten and the fall foliage show winds down, a quiet stand of conifers stands tall and stately and remain so through the winter. Edible plants with a cycle of ripening—plum trees, blueberries, artichokes, kale—can bear fruit in the same beds as ornamental plants. Plants can be left to hold their seedheads until wind or snow or foraging animals take them down. Users may find it therapeutic to draw or photograph the changing landscape.

Habitat gardens offer a rich sensory experience. They connect people to natural cycles and advance a healthy ecology. This approach to garden design transforms private traditional yards and public landscapes into places that attract birds, butterflies, bees, and other wildlife by providing them essential food and shelter. The gardens look and are allowed to behave like a natural landscape. The plants are pruned and shaped only as necessary for their health or to maintain views and paths through the site. Invasive species are removed, and native plants left to their natural patterns of growth and rest. Perennials are allowed to go to seed, providing food for birds, and leaves are left in place to compost and provide shelter and food for insects. Fertilizers are restricted to organic amendments. The layering of the native plants offers a deep sensory enrichment—aromatic, tactile, and subtly colorful. The seasonal change is accentuated when the plants are left in place to decompose and return to the earth. Often used in schools and community gardens, habitat gardens offer intergenerational learning opportunities and a sense of connection and belonging. The National Wildlife Federation offers a wildlife habitat certification program for qualifying gardens that have met the criteria by including the essential elements of food, water, and cover for wildlife and a place to raise their young.

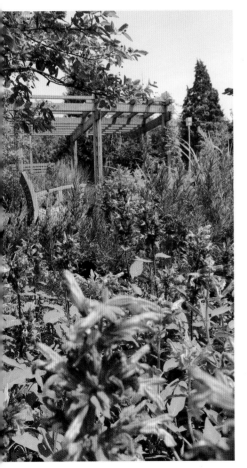

The right habitat attracts insects, birds, and other species that can delight and distract visitors from stressful experiences.

SITING PLANTS

In determining how to arrange plants, the designer is shaping spaces in the garden. When the plants are sequenced for a kind of visual musicality, the user is drawn in. Repeating drifts and masses of plants, flowering bulbs, and perennial groundcovers, for example, create a background for a focal specimen tree such as Japanese maple. The eye has a place to wander and to rest. Massings of singular plants, particularly stands of trees, are used to frame views and direct the user's gaze out of or into the garden. This visual journey provides both a sense of escape and restful focusing. Plants paired for contrast of color, tone, texture, movement, form, and size capture wonder and attention—for example, red-bronze coral bells with a chartreuse hebe, a crisply variegated hosta with a floriferous evergreen azalea, or quaking aspen behind a clipped boxwood hedge.

The designer uses a palette of plants to define, shape, and soften entries, rooms, and paths in the garden. In this process of softscaping, a room can be partitioned by climbing vines, a hedge of bamboo, or a grove of trees. In a similar way, unwanted views are screened or blocked. Vine-covered arbors and tree canopies are layered overhead to create shade and enclosure. An evergreen magnolia is not only beautiful, it stands out as a wayfinding landmark that people orient to as they move through the garden. If the goal is to maximize verdancy in the garden, the designer is restrained only by the site conditions for cultivation, availability of irrigation, and the outlay of costs for purchasing plants and maintaining them in the garden.

Finally, although the design team (or a consultant) will need experience in hydroponics and the commitment of facilities management if this site option is selected, hydroponic growing systems on rooftops might be an alternative when roof loads are adequate and the care and maintenance of the garden can be integrated into therapy programming. The plants, typically edibles, are grown in trays or tanks of nutrient-rich water. The advantage for those at risk of infection is that there is no contact with soil. Hydroponic gardens require a great deal of management and maintenance.

Rooftop Gardens

Therapeutic opportunities abound in rooftop garden spaces that offer pleasing views of city skylines, water, mountains, and changing skies. These absorbing vistas extend the feeling of escape beyond the boundaries of the rooftop and offer endless fascination and renewal. Those who for various reasons are unable to access a terra firma garden can breathe fresh air, feel the sun and soft breezes, and take in the garden scents. Rooftop spaces that are removed from the noise and commotion of urban streets offer a very quiet, private, and soothing experience for users experiencing stress, nausea, or intensive pain.

The elevation and openness of the rooftop also creates a microclimate and exposure to extremes of weather. The designer needs to mitigate for these conditions to make the garden comfortable and safe through most of the year. Hedges of bamboo, fastigate conifers such as Irish yew, and broadleaf evergreens such as California wax myrtle break and soften the wind. The planters can be insulated and heated. Built enclosures in the garden can have screens that are vine-planted or baffled and that are oriented to the prevailing winds. In regions prone to heavy wind, all built elements will require increased bracing and structural connections to ensure their stability and permanence. Securing all elements on a rooftop against wind uplift is critical, and any items not fastened down, such as furniture, will need to be heavy enough to counter wind velocities.

WEIGHT LOAD

In assessing a rooftop site for an existing building, the designers need to consult a structural engineer to understand the weight load capacity and the layout of the structural members. These restrictions will determine what can be designed, as measures to increase the load capacity are expensive. Two types of load calculations are made. A live load is the estimated weight of people and non-fixed elements such as therapy equipment and movable furniture. The dead load refers to the permanent elements such as walls, arbors, decks, or planters. "Combined load" is the live and dead loads, and this cannot exceed the structural capacity of the roof. Load is expressed in PSF (pounds per square foot), thus 60 PSF allows for 60 pounds per square foot of rooftop surface. Heavy elements such as mature trees are often sited on top of a load-bearing column, which may be capable of supporting additional weight. The floor plane is typically one of two systems that rest on top of the waterproofing membrane system, and this membrane needs to be preserved as structures are added. A wood or composition decking is attached to a wood-support framework or, alternatively, concrete pavers rest on plastic supports.

One strategy to reduce the dead load is to use lightweight planting mixes in the planters; these mixes are designed to not retain water, but because they are porous and deficient in nutrients, the planters will need frequent watering and fertilizer. Another is to use lightweight building materials. Polycarbonate, found in greenhouse structures, is much lighter than glass and can be used to cover arbors or pergolas. Water elements are typically designed with very shallow pools, and sheet flows are used instead of waterfalls.

SAFETY ISSUES

Containment barriers including walls, railings, panels, and screens are required by law to prevent users from falling off the roof and must meet local building codes. All these options offer adequate containment. Solid walls mitigate winds, but they block views. Railings do not impede the wind, and they interrupt visibility. Screens walls with solid or glass baffles deflect winds but also limit visibility. Glass panels buffer winds and allow unobstructed views. People with visual and perceptual challenges

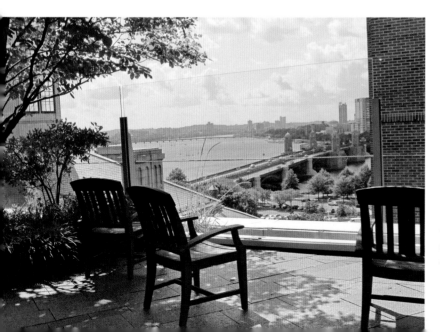

Glass panels ensure security, buffer wind, and preserve views.

may not be able to distinguish clear glass panels from the surrounding environment. Placing planters in front of the panels creates a safety barrier. For more open views and access, the panels can be mounted on low curb walls or fronted with kick rails, so those with reduced vision find a tactile cue to guide them.

Roof gardens are not always visible from inside the building, and they can be difficult to locate. Placing maps in the building lobby and signage in the corridors will facilitate wayfinding and access to the roof gardens. In older buildings, roof access was often gated and sized for maintenance personnel and may need to be enlarged or modified to accommodate current residents or patients. When the floor surface of the roof garden is lower than the interior access floor, the roof deck can be elevated.

MASKING MECHANICAL UNITS

The rooftop site often holds the mechanical units for the building, and they are unsightly and noisy. Roof vents circulate air into and out of the building; these are fixed once installed and need to be accessible for repair and replacement. Many existing units can be creatively integrated into a

At the Pete Gross House rooftop garden, a "living room," "porch/lounge," and "meditation/study" support the objective of a home-like retreat. Sightlines, screens, and plants ensure privacy and allow newcomers to tell if a room is already occupied.

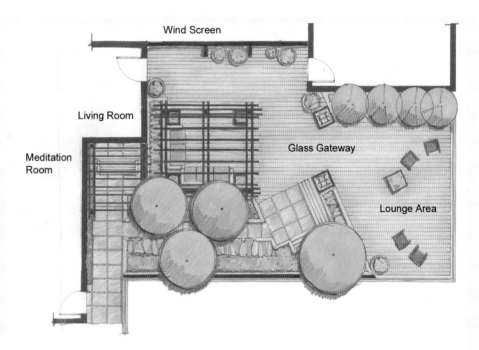

garden, as they were, for example, on the roof deck at Seattle's Pete Gross House, a temporary residence for people receiving cancer treatments. In this 1,200-square-foot project, the roof vents were aligned in two rows. Each fixed vent rose 18 inches above the floor plane and rotated with the wind. The designers synchronized the major garden structures—arbors, fencing, and screen panels—to join with the vent layout. Each vent was ornamented with a colored metal rectangular screen and cap. The vents in the main "living room" serve as end tables for the sofas and chairs, supporting bowls filled with succulents and river rocks, for tactile and visual interest; others became plinths for glass sculptures.

LEFT Each room is partitioned with deep blue painted wood screens and planters filled with aromatic herbs. The living room is enclosed and private with couches and chairs for reading, homework, meetings, and relaxed conversation. The roof vents go unnoticed.

RIGHT This small path serves as a transition space from the more active rooms to the meditative space. The chalkboard at its end was requested by resident children, so they could leave notes, create poems, and draw pictures for their peers.

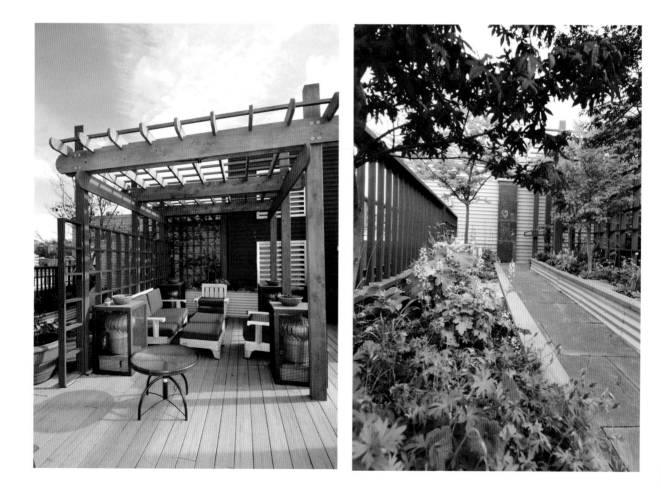

Lighting

Careful attention to lighting design will greatly enhance all the therapeutic values of the garden. Lighting promotes a sense of safety and extends the use of the garden in the evening and into the seasons of abbreviated daylight. Even if closed at sunset, subtle illumination can beautifully transform the garden for viewing at night.

A variety of lighting fixtures enables users to make their way through a garden by illuminating landmarks, entries, and pathways, by indicating edges, and by spotlighting trees, benches, and walls. Lighting is used to create ambience or mood and to delight; it can be very artful and dramatic, or calming and soothing.

Specific qualities of lighting are important to consider for people with mental illness, sensory challenges, or people with dementia, who may have distorted visual processing systems. Shadows or glare cast by lights may impede their ability to safely navigate through the garden. People with low vision, a condition that is untreatable with corrective lenses, surgery, or medication, also have particular lighting needs. The most common cause of low vision is age-related diseases of the eye such as macular degeneration, cataract, or glaucoma. When someone has low vision, being able to see curbs, curb cuts, changes in grade, and steps becomes very difficult, posing a significant safety risk in terms of trips, slips, and falls.

LIGHTING DESIGN PLAN

A lighting design plan for the garden will have both task lighting to spot wayfinding elements and ambient lighting to illuminate larger areas for circulation. Lighting needs to be constant and even along passageways. Downlighting is softer and easier on the eyes than uplighting. Uplighting can induce glare and cause temporary blindness, reducing a person's sense of stability and balance. At the same time some downlighting causes shadows, which can also be visually disruptive and confusing for people with mental health, dementia, or low vision issues. Additionally, downlighting can create distinct areas of high and low lighting, a challenge for eyes to adjust to while moving through the garden. An effective strategy is to pair low-level lighting like bollards with overhead peripheral lighting along paths; the shadowing effect, glare, and hot spots will be reduced where the illumination from both lighting fixtures crosses. Working closely with an occupational therapist with advanced training in low vision will be extremely helpful in selection and placement of appropriate lighting options for the therapeutic garden.

Lighting needs to be strategically installed along paths to guide users around curves and straightaways. In low-lighted areas, adults with low vision are more likely to have mobility issues, such as falls and decreased ambulation speed; they can veer off paths and collide with objects. LED lighting installed along a path's edging is an efficient way to keep people on track; it is a clear visual wayfinding cue. Lighting design will draw special attention to pathway intersections, changes in grade, drains, steps, ramps, and curbs. Information signage that is highly reflective, shiny, or plastic-coated can also create glare, making it hard to read. The use of matte finishes on signage and on all built structures will reduce glare and improve comfort and safety.

LIGHTING OPTIONS

A wide range of lights is available, including up and accents, in ground and well, path and spread, step and brick, and bollard and beacon lights. Each is designed for a specific purpose. Up and accent lights mounted in the ground are usually adjustable and used to highlight an object, such as a specimen tree or art work, or to wash a vertical plane. The units can be hidden behind vegetation; they should not be used near paths or plazas because, as they stick up above the ground surface, they could become a tripping hazard. Their lighting effects range from highly dramatic to soft and subtle. Ground and well lights sit flush or slightly raised above the ground plane and are used in paving, turf, or planting beds. Path and spread lights are low, usually with a hood that directs the light onto the ground plane; they are used to light paths and plazas and to flank entries and driveways. Step and brick lights are designed to sit flush with the face of a stair, ramp, or cheek wall; louvers or a hood direct the light downward to illuminate the paths and the bottom of the wall. Bollard and beacon lights rise up from the ground surface on bases; their columnar forms are also used to block access to a path or to separate cars and pedestrians.

Green Building Methods and Materials

To ensure users' health, the garden should be toxin-free. Those who have compromised immune systems are especially vulnerable to certain chemicals in the environment. It may also be meaningful to users if they understand that the designer's specified materials were sustainably harvested and manufactured. Green building methods and materials respect the environment and reduce the stresses on ecosystems. Stone and aggregates are durable building materials that in most regions are locally available. Wood should be sourced through (or designated as provided by) certified sustainable lumber suppliers. Both concrete and steel consume significant amounts of energy in the manufacturing and transportation processes. Each has many desirable qualities, including strength, durability, and long life span, but their judicious use will reduce the carbon footprint of the project. Treated lumber remains problematic. Toxic arsenic has been replaced with a preservative high in copper, which can adversely impact plants. Western juniper (*Juniperus occidentalis*), available in some regions, is used for retaining timbers, fencing, and decking; it is naturally resistant to rot, with a life span 30 years longer than other untreated western species, and requires no preservatives. In Europe, black locust (*Robinia pseudoacacia*) is widely used for exterior construction and prized for natural rot resistance and rapid growth. No doubt its use in the United States will increase as the lumber industry develops a market for it.

A wide selection of new and recycled materials including low-VOC paints, engineered wood products, rainwater harvesting systems, and porous paving products are available. Using plants to reduce runoff or treat water used in fountains and swimming pools is common in residential and public projects and can easily be integrated into therapeutic gardens. Solar and LED lights both reduce energy use, and drip irrigation increases efficiency while reducing water consumption. Creating spaces for human health should not damage or compromise the environment.

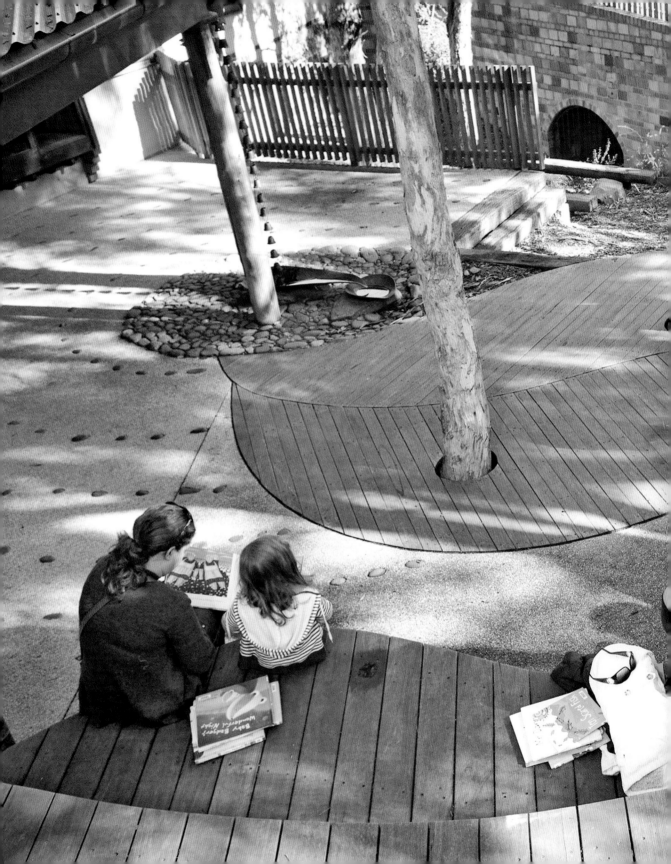

CHAPTER THREE
GARDENS FOR MOVEMENT AND PHYSICAL REHABILITATION

One area of focus in landscape architecture is receiving a lot of attention lately: the design of gardens meant to encourage children and adults with physical challenges to participate in gentle and safe exercise. When collaboratively and sensitively designed by a landscape architect and occupational therapist, the end result is an integrated, movement-focused therapeutic garden, one that seamlessly blends the knowledge of design with the knowledge of how the body functions. A successful movement garden is a space where children and adults of all ages and abilities feel confident to take risks, to challenge themselves to play and move.

Shared by a physical therapist: An elderly resident at a nursing facility had just arrived from the hospital after complications following a hip replacement. He did not want to be there. It was the last thing he anticipated, and he was terribly depressed. After he arrived and got settled in, his nurse aide took him on a tour. They went to the therapy clinic, where he met his OT and PT. As he looked around the clinic, he saw a glass door and through the door he saw, to his surprise, a courtyard garden, bustling with activity. It looked like therapists were working with patients on walking, climbing steps, wheeling, tending plants, and doing tabletop activities. Other residents were just strolling, puttering, and relaxing. The patient must have looked shocked, because the PT told him, "Oh, here we believe that health happens in the garden. If our patients want to have therapy outside and weather permits, we are there. It is up to each patient. But I have to tell you, most of them want to be outside. They say time passes faster, it is more fun, and it seems real. We like it better, too." The patient readily responded, "Count me in—when can I start my therapy, outside?"

Gardens for Children with Physical Challenges

Children with movement disorders often have some sort of developmental disability. A developmental disability occurs any time before age 22. Some examples of developmental disabilities include Down syndrome, cerebral palsy, spina bifida, and muscular dystrophy. More often than not, people with developmental disabilities have physical challenges that make movement difficult, but sometimes the physical challenge is only mild. Some may use wheelchairs or crutches to move around, and others will simply move slowly. There are no cures for any kind of developmental disability; they last a lifetime. For the purpose of design, reduced ability to move any part of the body independently can become a handicap, depending on the environmental context.

Seldom are children with movement disorders afforded the same outdoor experiences as their typically developing peers. Some of these children will learn differently than their peers, and some may simply be

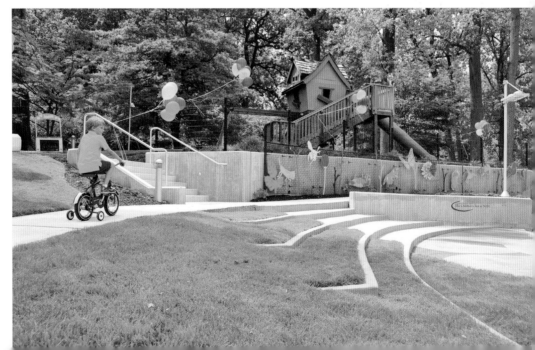

Designing for different levels of challenge lets children engage on their own terms, as here with three step configurations: shallow amphitheater steps, standard height steps, and steep steps up to the tree house.

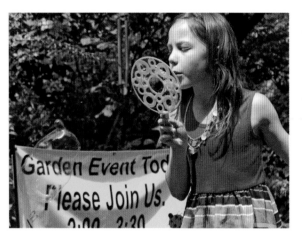

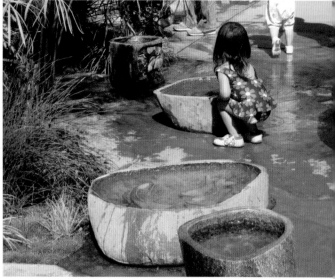

limited in the way that they move. Many do not have the opportunity to make their own choices; others do it for them. Some may, depending on the extent of their disability, be unable to direct their play. When such children are unable to experience outdoor play the same way their typically developing peers do, you actually see a downward spiraling effect and in many, a deep sense of isolation.

Outdoor play offers a substantial range of learning and developmental opportunities and benefits. Friendships are formed. Children learn to make choices and negotiate sharing toys and attention. They learn how to play in a group, to take turns, to solve problems, and to take risks (good ones, let us hope!). They learn to trust and challenge themselves. Being in nature inspires and supports creative fantasy and imaginative play. Outdoor play and movement go hand in hand. When environmental constraints limit a child's ability to make friends, play in a group, make choices, develop, move, and be creative, children may fall short of reaching their full potential. Therapeutic gardens can offer equitable directed and self-directed opportunities for children with movement challenges to experience the joys of being outside and in nature.

It is inappropriate to design therapeutic gardens that separate children with specific movement disorders from their typically developing peers. Separate but equal does not work; it only stigmatizes these children more than they already may be. Instead, think back to universal design, which reflects the needs of the widest range of people possible, regardless of age, ability, or preference. The overarching goal when designing for

LEFT Creative play often has active, movement-oriented components associated with it.

RIGHT For most children, the allure of water is irresistible. Touching, splashing, pouring, measuring, and displacing water is fun, keeps children moving, and is educational. Seemingly simple innocuous bins filled with water fascinate this child.

children with movement challenges is to provide ample opportunities to make choices, develop friendships, be creative, and to move. The design should be child-centered, featuring elements that hold universal appeal for children.

Not surprisingly, general recommendations for designing therapeutic gardens for children with movement disorders share some common characteristics with their adult counterparts. It may not be feasible to incorporate all the universal design concepts into one therapeutic garden. Occupational, physical, and speech therapists, parents and siblings, teachers, and most importantly, the children themselves are the best resources for prioritizing what will be included. Using this type of participatory design process will lead to more responsive results that meet the participant's needs and therefore be more likely to succeed.

Optimal adjacencies to a proposed or existing building (school, clinic, hospital, or community center) is a primary consideration. The closer the garden is to the building, the easier it will be to access. It will be more likely to be used, especially if time is an issue, as with scheduled therapy sessions.

A level courtyard deck adjacent to a neighborhood library is an ideal place for children to choose to be active or sit quietly and be read to by caring adults. No stigma is attached to either choice.

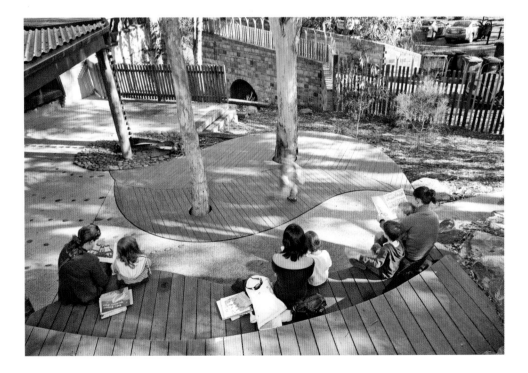

CLOSER LOOK

Kennedy Krieger Institute

Mahan Rykiel Associates worked collaboratively with the clinical therapy staff at the Kennedy Krieger Institute to design and complete a half-acre therapy garden at the new outpatient center in Baltimore, Maryland. Serving the needs of children with complex brain disorders, staff at Kennedy Krieger recognize the value of engaging children with outdoor experiences. The garden was designed as a series of rooms specifically to complement the indoor therapeutic capacities. Varied textures, elevation changes, spatial scale, and sensory-rich elements, like a labyrinth, stones, plantings to explore, and central lawn, are linked via an interactive wheelchair-height water runnel. Guided by their therapists, children work on goal-oriented mobility, sensory, cognitive, and motor skills as they explore and traverse the garden's varied paving surfaces as a means to replicate what they encounter in the community. They play and reap the physical, emotional, and spiritual benefits of being outside. The therapy garden has achieved its goals. From the outset of the project, it brought together the skills and knowledge bases of design and therapy to create a model outdoor therapy garden. It is a child-centered place where engaging in therapy is a joyful experience for the children, their therapists, and their families.

A water runnel sweeps along the garden's perimeter wall. Set at a height suitable for children in wheelchairs, it beckons to be touched.

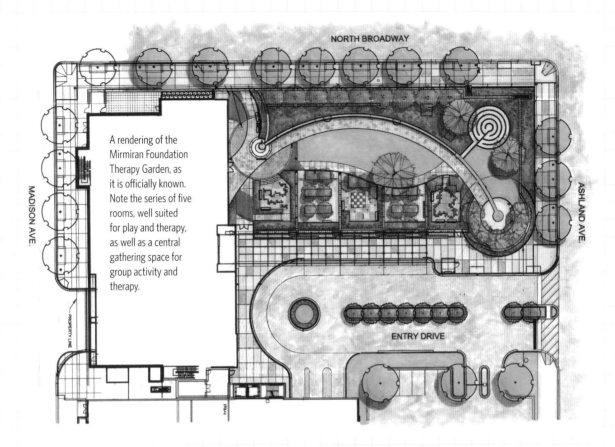

NORTH BROADWAY

MADISON AVE.

ASHLAND AVE.

A rendering of the Mirmiran Foundation Therapy Garden, as it is officially known. Note the series of five rooms, well suited for play and therapy, as well as a central gathering space for group activity and therapy.

PROPERTY LINE

ENTRY DRIVE

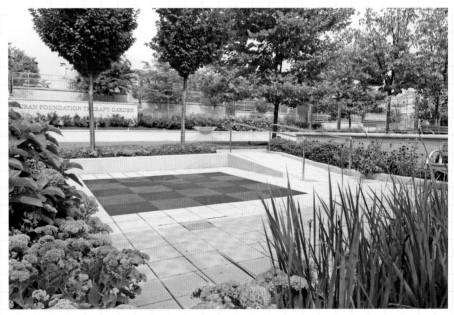

A low slope ramp with parallel railing and vari-colored and -surfaced paving materials are useful rehabilitation elements for children working on mobility skills.

If this is not possible, a clear and unobstructed path from the building to the garden must be maintained. When accessing the garden, make the journey a pleasant one. Whimsical or kinetic sculpture is fun to look at and can become meeting places or fun stops along the way. There is no stigma in stopping to look at sculpture, when in fact you are really taking a rest. A raised waterway for children to dangle their fingers in and follow along the journey to the garden, whether they get there on foot or via a wheelchair, enhances the play experience. No matter the distance or size, getting to and moving within the garden is exercise.

PARTICIPATORY DESIGN WITH SPECIAL-NEEDS CHILDREN

Even the youngest end users must remain at the center of therapeutic garden design. One very simple and successful way to involve children in a participatory design process is to invite them and the significant adults in their lives to a design charette. Provide the young garden users with their own "grown-up" paper and markers for sharing their ideas. Ask the children (first!) to draw their best and most special ideas for their perfect outdoor garden play space on sheets of paper hung on walls and set on table tops. Parents, therapists, and teachers should be available to guide the children but not to direct them. Be patient; some may have trouble conveying their thoughts visually.

Some children with movement disorders will be wheelchair users and may have trouble writing in ways that are familiar to you. Be sure to include a request for parents, occupational therapists, or teachers to bring whatever special writing tools a child needs. Asking children who use wheelchairs to draw on a sheet of paper hung on a wall will be uncomfortable, if not impossible, as they will have to be positioned sideways to reach the paper and draw. Providing options, to draw either on a vertical surface (wall) or a horizontal surface (table), shows a deeper level of understanding of and empathy for the complex needs of all children.

The optimal way to review the charette activities is, with written permission, to videotape it. It is hard to simultaneously observe, listen, take notes, and respond to all the ideas that will be flowing. Your collaborative designer/occupational therapy team can review the video documentation and better understand the ideas before translating them into a design.

Another successful way to gather input from children, as with their adult counterparts, is to create photos of preference activities. A deck of cards, each featuring an image of an element or activity, can be sorted by the children into two piles, like or dislike. This can also be accomplished with image boards, where photos or drawings are grouped around a theme such as edible gardens, fun plant choices, or play activities. The children are given sticker dots, red or green, to indicate that they like or dislike the image they are posting it by. The patterns and preferences thus revealed will inform the design.

DESIGN CONSIDERATIONS

Incorporate elements that enable children to make choices, to decide if playing with a large or small group meets their needs. In these special gardens, whatever children choose to do is safe and whenever they choose to do it is okay. Because children with movement disorders tend to have fewer opportunities to make individual choices and experience autonomy, a design that offers choices is paramount.

Pots filled with textural plants that beckon to be touched are also important. Placing a bench proximal to these points of interest provides informal resting spots for children whose endurance is low and can also encourage socialization. The rest spots should allow those in wheelchairs to pause and socialize with those using the benches without blocking the path. Not only can one be seen at the rest spots, you can view others wandering by.

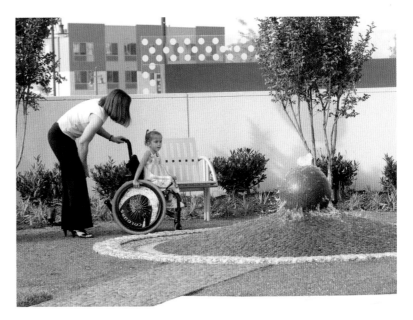

Stopping along the way to gaze at a strategically placed feature of interest eliminates the stigma of needing a place to rest.

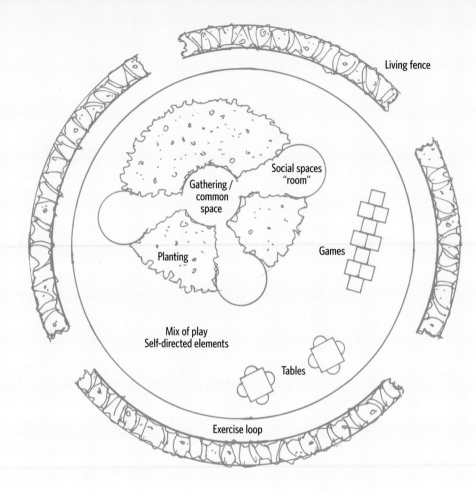

Living fence

Gathering / common space

Social spaces "room"

Planting

Games

Mix of play
Self-directed elements

Tables

Exercise loop

Designing designated areas in the garden for specific movement purposes encourages activity and exploration. Ringed by a perimeter exercise loop, the garden becomes an inviting place to move through and explore.

Conceptually, movement garden design can be understood as a series of interconnected concentric experiences that provide options for children to make choices about where and what they want to do. With this type of design, the innermost circle, the common space, is flanked by a series of smaller social spaces, which are nestled within the outer exercise zone, and wrapped within a surrounding enclosure.

Children, not the design, should direct the play. A simple, flat, grassy central common becomes a multipurpose space for children to play in medium to large groups. A mesh underlay that provides extra surface rigidity will make it easier for children in wheelchairs to traverse the space. Keep it simple—soft grass and a few raised mounds for play make for imaginative play. Design adequate room at the bottom of these knolls so that their momentum is stopped before children enter a pathway. Some children will climb up and roll down them, and some who cannot move on their own may simply enjoy having an adult carry them to the top and help them place their bare feet on the soft grass so they can wiggle their toes.

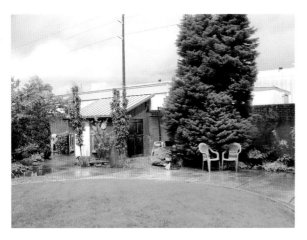

Open grassy areas in a garden serve it well; they are ideal places for spontaneous directed and self-directed active play and movement.

The small nooks or rooms offset from the common space should have wide interconnected walkways. This is ideal for adults to supervise children at play. A short, 12-inch hedge of fragrant herbs offers a sense of separation between the nooks and an olfactory experience, while still maintaining a 360-degree sightline for adult supervision. Child-sized furniture and wheelchairs can be tucked into these socialization nooks, and a nine-foot turning radius defined by the hedge enables a wheelchair to easily turn around. Create multiple entries to all other nooks, and ring these socialization spaces with a "trike track"—a wide, paved pathway for children to exercise, practice walking skills, pedal a tricycle, wheel a chair around, and engage in a diverse range of movements. The track should be made of appropriate material that will cushion a fall, preventing abrasions and impact-related injuries. At the Camborne Nursery School in Cornwall, Westley Design installed a highly popular multisurface universal access trike track for children to pedal, wheel, or wander around at their own pace and terms. What kind of movement will this very simple garden design encourage? The garden provides children opportunities to reach up and bend down, to stand and sit, to walk, run, march, skip, roll their bodies or wheelchairs, or climb.

How can challenge be infused into this kind of a garden? Those grassy mounds should be of varying heights, slopes, and widths to accommodate a range of skills and abilities. Taking laps around the trike trail is a graded challenge: day one, a child travels a quarter of the way around with help, and perhaps by day 45 that same child can go halfway around—on his or her own. Planters at different heights tempt children to reach up or bend down to explore the plants, thus encouraging movement and offering a chance to practice balance skills. Vibrant, variously textured outdoor children's play mats can be hung along the fence at varying heights for a child to reach up or down to touch—another balance and movement challenge.

If a more structured movement garden is considered with additional destinations (elements), one can be a simple obstacle course all children can navigate. The course may include a slalom that is created by planting trees six feet apart (to accommodate wheelchairs) for children and adults to weave in between, a bridge climb (1:30 ramp to platform to ramp) over

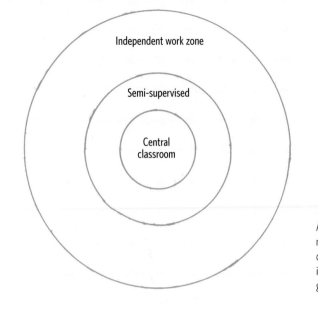

A concentric ring design concept maximizes movement opportunities and encourages children to expand their skills and move to increasingly more challenging areas in the garden.

a dry creek bed, and a terrain path (crushed gravel transitioning to ADA matting, transitioning to smooth paving). These elements, on their own or grouped as a single course, help improve movement and balance skills. Curved paths with clearly demarcated edging make the journey more interesting and challenging. Wider paths enable people to travel in different directions or together at the same time.

Other destination ideas are a simple hedge maze, 18 to 24 inches high, that does not restrict sightlines for supervision, or a multilevel sandbox with retractable covers to restrict unwanted animals. The multiple levels mean children in wheelchairs can play side by side with those standing or sitting. A lift, similar to those used at therapeutic swimming pools, or a transfer deck can be installed so children who are unable to lower themselves to the ground can experience a full-body sandbox play experience. Swings are also an all-important feature. Many freestanding swings work well for children with all types of movement challenges.

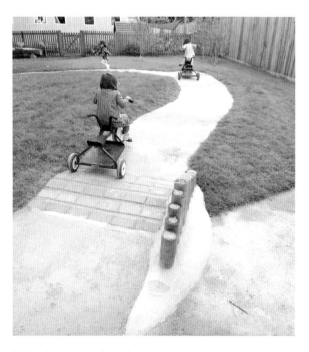

Ringing the perimeter of a garden, a level trike track formed of various surfaces provides multiple opportunities for children to run, walk, and ride at their own paces.

Gardens for Adults with Physical Challenges

Just like children, adults with physical challenges deserve to experience the benefits of a therapeutic garden and partake in gentle exercise. These types of gardens are usually found at healthcare facilities as an extension of a rehabilitation clinic where therapy goals are addressed. They may also be installed at community parks, elder care facilities, and senior centers. Adults with movement-related diseases or conditions like arthritis, multiple sclerosis, cancer, stroke, spinal cord injury, and heart disease may benefit most from movement-oriented therapeutic gardens. If the garden is being designed as a rehabilitation garden at a healthcare or senior living facility, working closely with the therapists ensures that elements and concepts that are unique to meet the needs of that facility will be included. Designing a safe and inviting all-season place for adults with

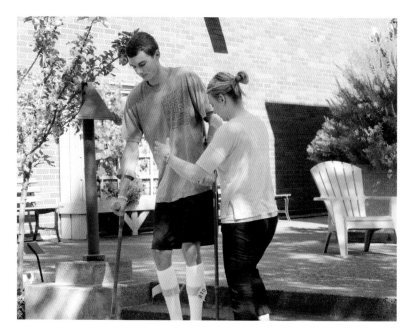

For many, not just young adults, rehabilitation outdoors in a controlled environment is highly motivating.

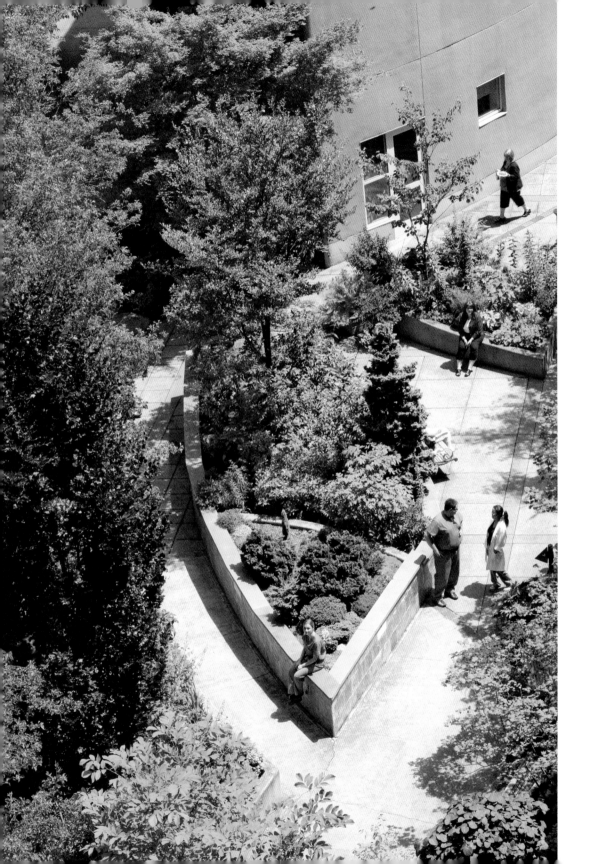

OPPOSITE At the Stenzel Healing Garden at Legacy Good Samaritan Medical Center in Portland, Oregon, seating walls stand ready to accommodate staff, community members, and patients with decreased balance and endurance.

RIGHT This therapeutic garden provides adults with developmental disabilities an opportunity to learn the vocational skill of garden maintenance. The colorful kinetic sculpture is a positive distraction, visually stimulating, and often triggers a conversation.

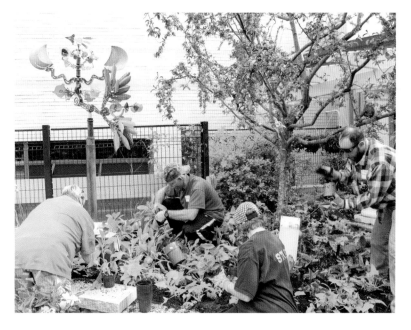

physical challenges to move and heal outdoors is highly achievable. The aim remains for the space to be rich with physical, visual, and sensory interactions, whether it is on the ground or on a rooftop (see chapter 2 for more on rooftop gardening).

DESIGN CONSIDERATIONS

Therapeutic gardens for adults with physical challenges share commonalities with children's gardens. They need to offer choice and reinforce sense of control. When possible, especially if the garden is intended to be an extension of the rehabilitation clinic, adjacency will increase its usability. Views into the garden can also be motivating.

Design wide and curving paths with ample shade and seating every 10 to 15 feet; this affords those who need it a place to stop and re-energize without worrying about making it to the next rest spot. These rest spots should be set back from paths so wheeled mobility devices can tuck in without impeding traffic.

With age, many people experience joint pain and limitations in movement. Seating with armrests is critical because it helps people rise from and gently ease down into the seat. Adirondack chairs are attractive and

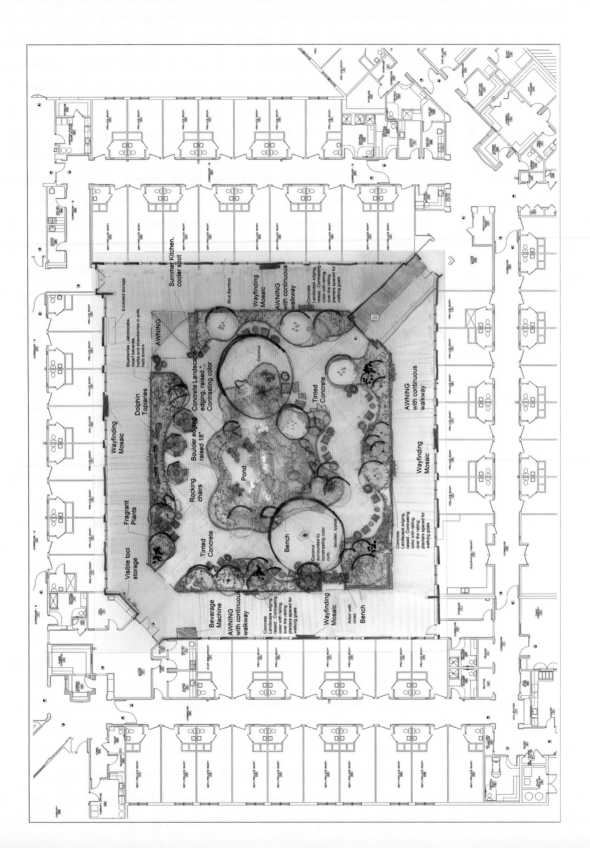

Enclosed storage

Summer Kitchen, cooler spot

Blueberries, Jaboticaba, dwarf bananas, herbs and strawberries in pots, herb towers

Blue Bamboo

AWNING

Wayfinding Mosaic

AWNING with continuous walkway

Concrete Landscape edging, raised. Contrasting color. Raised. Contrasting color with railing over the railing planters spaced for walking goals

Dolphin Topiaries

Coconut

Boulder edging raised 18"

Concrete Landscape edging, raised. Contrasting color.

Tinted Concrete

Wayfinding Mosaic

Fragrant Plants

Rocking chairs

Pond

AWNING with continuous walkway

Visible tool storage

Tinted Concrete

Wayfinding Mosaic

Coconut surrounded by contrasting color curb boulder, typical

Concrete Landscape edging, raised. Contrasting color with railing over the railing planters spaced for walking goals

Beverage Machine

AWNING with continuous walkway

Concrete Landscape edging, raised. Contrasting color with railing over the railing planters spaced for walking goals

Wayfinding Mosaic

Bench

Arbor with vines

Bench

OPPOSITE A rendering of a senior living courtyard garden. The center focuses on deep connections with nature and then progresses outward to active areas, demonstrating how varying levels of challenge and interaction can be integrated into a single design.

iconic in gardens, but they are not a good option for those with limited movement capacities. They tend to be low to the ground, and the reclined back makes it difficult to transition from a sitting to standing position. Chairs with upright backs are easier to get up from. People are not of equal size or shape, so seating options that will serve the tallest and smallest users well are recommended.

For those who want to track distance walked, integrate subtle distance markers at strategic points along the paths. Making pathways measured walking trails enables users to partake of outdoor exercise in a controlled environment. Measured walking trail signage is installed at several of the Legacy Health gardens in Portland, Oregon; the signage includes information about walking distances, encouraging words about the benefits of walking as exercise, and curiosity-enticing clues for what to look for in the journey around the garden.

Paths must be free of debris and slip-resistant; every possible precaution to avoid falls along their course must be taken. There is a strong case for tinted concrete paths, which minimize glare. But here is a twist: if you are designing a therapeutic garden at a rehabilitation, healthcare, or elder care facility, consider a discussion with staff occupational and physical therapists and risk-management personnel about the merits of installing

At most any stage in life, moving physical rehabilitation outdoors can lead to patients and staff feeling greater satisfaction with the process. Red flowers and feeders along this course mean hummingbirds may just be added to the healthy mix.

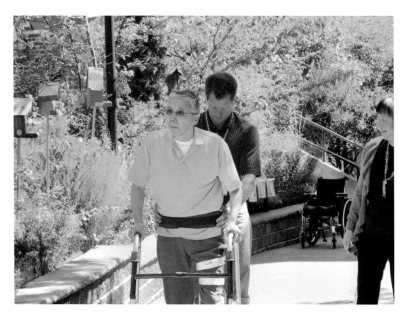

a cobblestone or reflexology trail on one subpath. A study found that 60- to 92-year-olds who regularly walked on cobblestones actually had better balance than those who did not (Li et al. 2005). In the design world, this presents a risk-tolerance dilemma. Cobblestones are difficult to walk on and pose a slip, trip, and fall hazard. In order to reduce falling over the long haul, knowing that those who regularly walk on them develop better balance skills than those who do not may justify the risks. For the health and safety of the users, cobblestone installation needs to be a collaborative decision made with experts who work directly with older adults.

Railings should flank all paths. Not only are they very important safety features, they often function as impromptu exercise/rehabilitation elements. They are

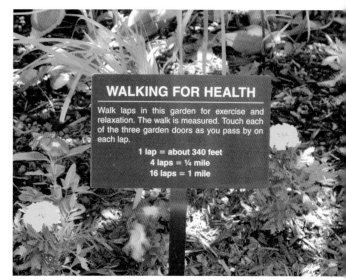

TOP For those tracing progress in a formal goal-directed ambulation program, easy-to-read signage denoting distances and destinations in the garden is important.

BOTTOM Handrails are seamlessly integrated into the design, providing safe passage for users while not compromising aesthetics.

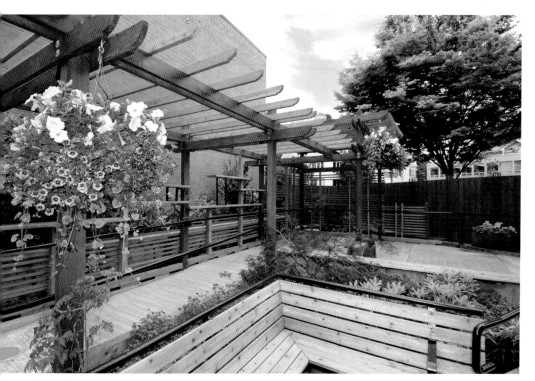

convenient supportive elements to grasp and practice push-ups, knee bends, leg lifts, and foot and ankle stretches. Users can stand parallel to the railing and gaze into the garden. Railings, when designed properly, can be aesthetic features and certainly should not look cold and institutional. Bright color contrast is important for aging eyes, and painting or powder-coating the rails a vivid color may both aid in wayfinding and complement your color scheme. When color and material is incorporated into other elements of the garden, the railing will feel less disconnected and more harmonious with the overall design and become a language of detailing instead of a functional intervention. Hanging planters above or adjacent to the railings at set increments allows users to track their walking distance; it is also an invitation to stop to tend and enjoy the planter boxes.

Railings enhance physical use of the garden and provide psychological reassurance for those who might not otherwise venture into the garden. At Theda Clark Medical Center in Neenah, Wisconsin, the HGA design team worked collaboratively with the hospital's therapy and nursing team from the beginning to design, among other elements, a much-requested at-grade footbridge. An earlier version of the plan proposed an open water feature, which included a bridge and a zero-depth entry to allow for direct interaction with water. This raised maintenance concerns; but the design team understood the overall therapeutic benefits of including the sight and sound of water, and did not want to eliminate this element. As a result, HGA explored a dry water feature option. With this design, running water is visible, recirculating through the spillway element. Exploring this option with therapists and facilities management led to a low-maintenance solution and provided an important therapy element. Working together, they developed a spillway bridge with a detailed railing system to support the needs of the therapy team.

A movement garden for adults contains a level central gathering space surfaced with rubberized resilient playground matting and multiple access routes connecting to a primary path. Instead of leaving this gathering area open, as suggested for a children's movement garden, an adult fitness zone may be more

Collaborative design leads to low-maintenance, high-quality solutions—in this case, a detailed railing system on an at-grade footbridge.

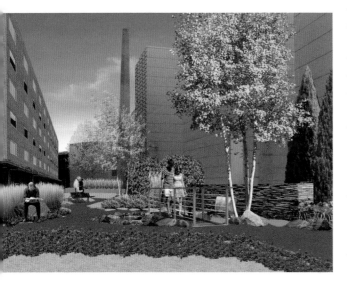

appropriately incorporated into this space. Outdoor movement transforms dreary exercise into a multisensory experience that encourages balance, strengthening, and social interaction.

An adult fitness zone is essentially a gym moved outdoors. This equipment is universally designed and specifically fabricated for outdoor use to meet a wide range of people's needs. Leaving at least 10 feet of space between each piece of equipment enables people to pass by without impeding someone else's workout. If a fitness zone is not a possibility, consider using the centralized exercise area for yoga or tai chi. Other areas of the garden incorporate a variety of walking surfaces that offer choice and options for those who wish to challenge themselves with more rigorous exercise options. Multilevel drinking fountains, shade, ample seating for rest breaks and observation, and a handicapped restroom are amenities that enhance the comfort level and ensure that users will visit and stay longer in the garden.

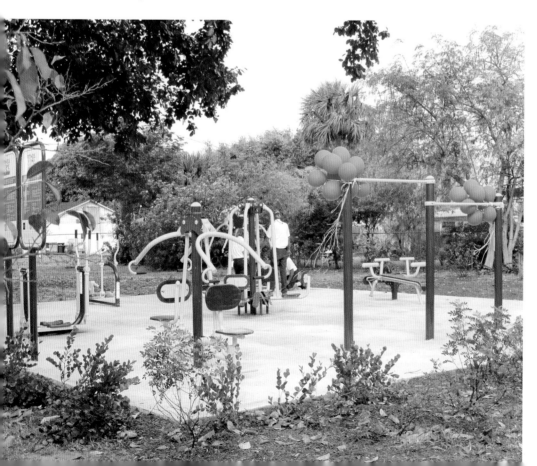

Installing a universally designed public outdoor fitness zone is a cost-effective way to build community and encourage movement and exercise.

Gardens for Children with Cancer

Therapeutic garden design for children with cancer share both commonalities and differences with the gardens just discussed. The most important commonality is to offer choice and enhance sense of control for children (and their families) to do, to move, to be, and to feel whole.

Children diagnosed with cancer usually begin life healthy and develop in a typical sequence, and parents dream that their child will always be healthy and thrive. Cancer, a dreaded diagnosis, may elicit an overwhelming sense of fear and helplessness in parents when they learn their child has it. A therapeutic garden may become the place for all burdens and fears to dissipate, even if for just a few moments.

Children undergoing cancer treatment, like their adult counterparts, are vulnerable to infection because their immune systems are highly suppressed. This vulnerability translates into periods of isolation when the children may be unable to go outside or interact with other people unless proper infection control measures are taken. Isolation, a disconnection from people and nature, leads to loneliness, depression, confusion, and anger. In an ideal world, children too ill to go into the therapeutic garden would have visual access, as research shows that even passive views of nature can improve health. Designers should consider siting therapeutic gardens within an enclosed rooftop, courtyard, building lobby, or terrace so it can be viewed by those unable to go outside. Many healthcare facilities have stringent infection control rules, so even indoor gardens separated by glass or limited to a rolling plant trolley may not be possible unless the plants are grown in soil-less medium. A clear viewing room for children to go to and feel as if they are surrounded by nature is buffering and offers one way to bring the healing effects of nature into their lives.

Children's therapeutic gardens should convey hope, peace, optimism, and connection. Children often respond to imagery and humor; elements that spark whimsy and curiosity are counterpoints to the fear and uncertainty connected with their illness. At the St. Louis Children's Hospital Olson Family Garden designed by Herb Schaal, all these considerations are incorporated into a vibrant garden space used for therapy, recreation, and relaxation. The garden has a wheelchair-accessible kaleidoscope, water

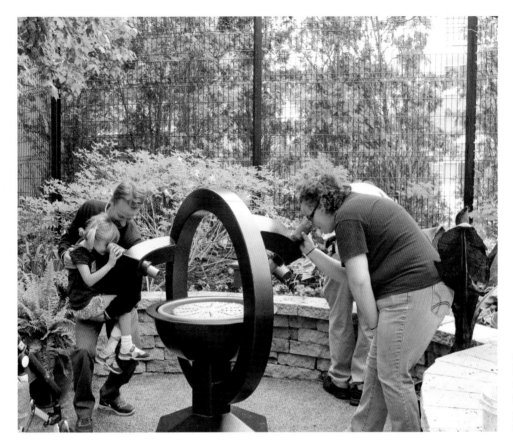

A universally designed kaleidoscope is a wonderful distraction for all pediatric patients and those who love them.

features, an interactive spinning stone, nooks to snuggle into and gaze out over the city, a bridge, ample open and shaded seating, and a profusion of plantings that, in partnership with clients at an area center for adults with developmental disabilities, are changed with the seasons.

DESIGN CONSIDERATIONS

A garden designed for children with cancer must include an abundance of shade created by sails, trees, umbrellas, covered structures, or green screens to protect sensitive skin from the sun's harmful rays. Budgeting for mature trees and other structural shade elements is essential. Plantings must be free of thorns or sharp edges and have zero toxicity. Because sense of smell is altered during chemotherapy, reconsider the use of highly aromatic plants. As for the other senses, select plants that are eye-catching (towering sunflowers), or make fun sounds in the wind (bamboo stalks clicking together), or are fun to touch (lamb's ears, mimosa, wooly thyme).

OPPOSITE TOP Including ample and comfortable seating for all users is an important consideration in therapeutic garden design. Finding an inviting place to sit and feel cared about can ease the anxiety associated with medical treatment.

OPPOSITE BOTTOM Well-maintained soft grassy areas invite spontaneous play and movement, especially when they are furnished with an engaging palette of sunny flowers, unexpected art, and astonishing topiary.

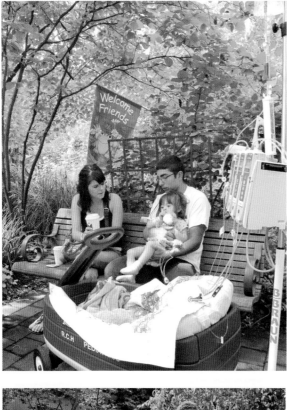

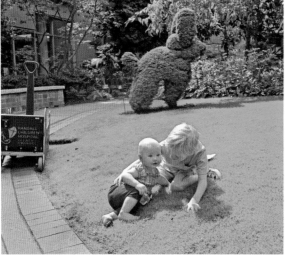

All paths must be smooth and relatively flat with joint spaces not to exceed ⅛ inch or be sealed flush with the surrounding paving to prevent an IV pole, cane, or other medical equipment from getting stuck between the pavers. Falls risk must be minimized, and a resilient impact-resistant surfacing should be considered as an option.

To support emotional health, create small private gathering spaces for prayer and reflection. Pergolas planted with flowering vines or gourds, tiki huts, or other regionally specific shelters can accomplish this. Reduce or counteract intrusive noise transmissions, perhaps by incorporating gentle wind chimes or natural elements like rustling ornamental grasses or bamboos. Include ample space for tables and wheelchairs or gurneys to access these shady, quiet zones, and furnish them with movable chairs for children and adults to rearrange for their needs. Design unobtrusive storage to hold table games, paper and pens, bottles of water, and tissues; including passive diversions like games and sundries will make quiet spaces feel more homelike and comfortable.

In the garden children should be given the opportunity to experience a genuine sense of getting away and relief. Designing for escape as a counterpoint to the institutional feel of a medical setting should be embedded in any therapeutic garden. Natural lighting instead of fluorescent, breezes instead of air conditioning, gentle sounds of rustling leaves or simple quietude instead of machine-made noises, and plants to view and touch provide this counterpoint. Some plantings should be close enough to touch while others may be more distant; distant landscape provides soft fascination and accentuates the depth field, conveying a sense of expansion and escape. The garden should be as green and lush as possible, so the experience of place is nurturing and comforting. It is also appropriate and beneficial to incorporate whimsy into the garden.

CLOSER LOOK

Beacon Hill Nursery School

Beacon Hill Nursery School, tucked into the Boston neighborhood of the same name, serves students aged two to six. There was little existing space for outdoor play nearby, so when the city deeded the adjacent 2,500-square-foot city playground to the school, executive director Lucinda Ross was delighted. After researching the effects of limited exposure to nature on child development, she retained landscape

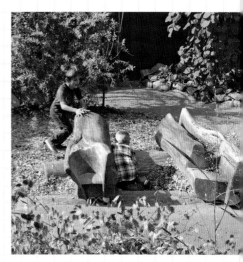

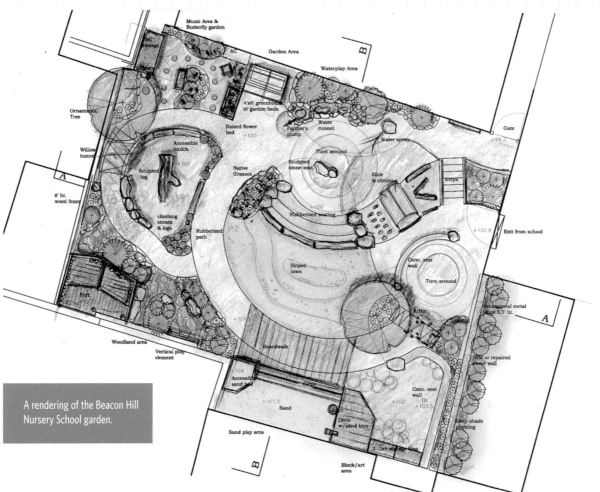

A rendering of the Beacon Hill Nursery School garden.

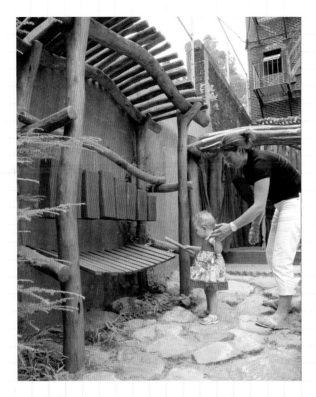

design firm Johansson Design Collaborative and Holly D. Ben-Joseph, landscape architect and conceptual design consultant, to design a natural playscape. Although no children at the time needed it as such, the nursery school playground was intentionally designed to be accessible, and children are free to select their activities within it. They build dams and manipulate the water cascading down a river rock runnel lined with movable rocks; they roll down or crawl up a grassy knoll. They can dig and carve canals in the sandbox and then fill them with water from the nearby hand pump, or sit in the amphitheater for outdoor learning and then zip down the adjacent slide when class is not in session. Swings and climbing ropes, proven favorites to include in any movement garden, are included. The nature curriculum at Beacon Hill inspires children to learn more about the world around them, and their place within it. Their school's playscape recaptures some of the magic most of us remember from our youth—magic that begins with creating a world through play and nature.

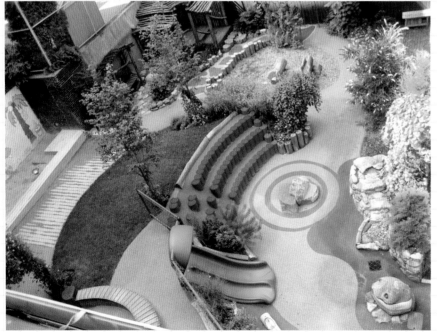

OPPOSITE TOP Vertically and horizontally oriented logs of various height and widths present as a fun and spontaneous balance element, encouraging imaginative play and movement. Whether this is leapfrog or hide and seek is anyone's guess.

TOP With guidance from a teacher, even the youngest children can risk traversing bumpy terrain and then challenge their balance further by striking a wood xylophone with a mallet.

BOTTOM An aerial view of the Beacon Hill Nursery School garden.

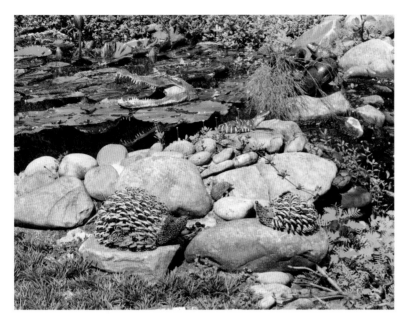

Whimsical sculpture provides positive distraction and a focal point to redirect attention outward.

Vertical gardens planted with highly saturated flowers evoke joy. Children will be unable to resist touching the plants, installed at various heights, even if they have to stand on tiptoes to do so, and they cannot help but laugh at plants that live in smelly old boots or some other fun repurposed object, like a washtub. If facility procedures allow, a rack of child-sized garden tools and a scrub brush next to the tub will invite young patients to tend the garden and clean the outside of the tub, as a formal or informal rehabilitation element. Sculpture should be easy to understand and relate to; it need not necessarily be comical and overly juvenile but easily identifiable. For example, in the Leichtag Family Healing Garden at Rady Children's Hospital San Diego, sea stars and other sea animal sculptures reference the nearby Pacific Ocean; and in the Prouty Garden at Boston Children's Hospital, a bear, a frog, and birds all native to the region quietly hide in little nooks just waiting for that curious explorer to find them.

Stone retaining wall niches provide wonderful opportunities to tuck in treasures and trailing herbs. Tiny porcelain fairy figurines dance on a garden wall in the children's garden at Kanapaha Botanical Gardens in Gainesville, Florida, awaiting discovery by curious children and their families. For those seeking more

Sculpture that references the local area links a garden to the wider environment. Child-sized ride-on and climbable sculpture increases the appeal of any movement garden meant for children, and bright colors and touchable features only add to their charm.

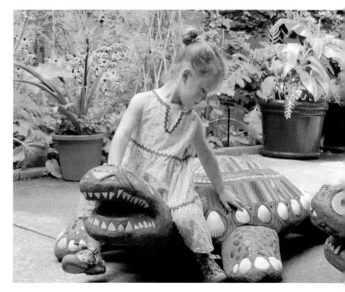

active things to do, a treasure hunt is great fun and educational as well, as children look for specific plants, trees, and other elements tucked within the garden. Guided with a map and photos of what is to be found, children are engaged and kept moving. It is also a welcome distraction from diagnosis, illness, or treatment.

Brightly colored perimeter walls disguise their primary purpose and can be designed to blend into the garden's purpose and theme. They can also serve as a wayfinding element. Ceramic tile mosaics can make the journey along a perimeter path more interesting by telling a story to young patients who badly need the distraction; they are also appealingly

A colorful nautical theme designed by clients was installed along a perimeter wall at the Lighthouse of Broward in Fort Lauderdale, Florida.

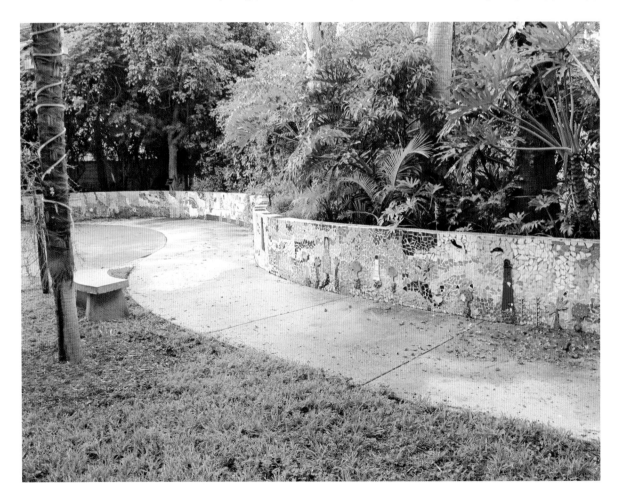

touchable for people with residual vision as well as those with sight.

Placing unexpected objects like chimes or fancy bird cages off to the side or in the upper plane of vision—in trees, light standards, or arbors—invites children to look up or permits children in gurneys or wheelchairs to see within their restricted lines of sight. Think about how vines can be integrated into your design. Train them to dangle down and create natural curtains. Orient them sideways for children to slide their hands along as they walk or are wheeled through the paths in the garden. Walls of corn, grains, or bamboo can be space definers. Interpretive signage transmits a deeper awareness about the plantings, their role in medicine, and the garden itself. Use highly contrasting background coloring and lettering, pictures, an audio button, and Braille on these signs.

For designers, water features again present a quandary as they pose a high infection control risk, the splash and runoff creates slippery surfaces, and water quality can be contaminated by animals. Yet children are inexorably drawn to water. There are ways that the qualities of water without the actual water can be incorporated into the therapeutic garden. A "creek" lined with lovely pieces of blue and green sea glass meanders through the Carter School Sensory Garden in Boston; it functions as a wayfinding element of sorts and a point of tactile fascination as sea glass is smooth and pleasant to touch. Another option is a recirculating water feature that is inaccessible to curious children but designed to provide visual and auditory appeal, like a water-spitting dragon or gargoyle. These types of elements are fun, whimsical, and distracting and could easily become the topic of many silly stories for children to share and act out with their caregivers.

Creating movement gardens for children with cancer requires creativity, empathy, sensitivity, respect, common sense, collaboration, and research. Working closely with the hospital staff is critically important; they can tell you what will give children and their families much-needed respite, and what will allow them to forget their immediate burdens and escape into a natural world. Children with cancer are very ill, but they are still children: these therapeutic gardens should abound with and inspire optimism.

Gardens for Children with Obesity

Childhood obesity remains a serious public health issue. As of 2012, according to the Centers for Disease Control and Prevention, 18 percent of children and 21 percent of adolescents in the United States were obese. One explanation is that children are not getting enough exercise. Many have little or no safe outside place, or feel unwelcomed to play. For children with obesity, movement gardens that encourage gentle exercise can help to reverse this trend. These gardens are not designed exclusively for children with obesity: the stigma attached to being sent to a "special garden" would defeat the purpose.

DESIGN CONSIDERATIONS

A high degree of sensitivity is required when designing gardens to meet the needs of children who are obese. Consider how the garden can be designed with universal features to encourage extra subtle movement opportunities for all children, including those with obesity. Additional movement equates to exercise. If seating has a movement element associated with it, children will unconsciously be using their bodies. Rocking

Slides are obvious, but any element that requires movement to activate—bench swings, gliders, bouncy toys—offers subtle exercise opportunities.

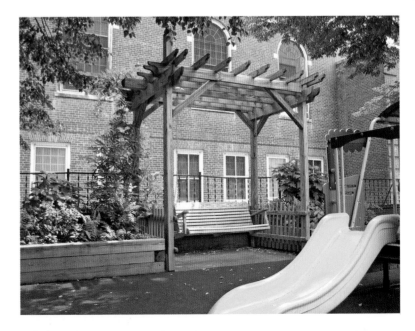

chairs and bench swings are a perfect example. We are not suggesting setting out a row of grandma's rocking chairs but rather something akin to carved-out logs that have a rocking mechanism. Spring-based seats or a stack of tires lashed together and set on their sides offer a simple opportunity for children who are sitting to instead be moving.

Seating that is two inches lower than standard children's chair height means that children have to work just a bit harder to sit down and get back up (visit communityplaythings.com for chair height guidelines). Seating with and without armrests and differently angled backs offers varied sets of movement challenges. This is the time to bring out the iconic Adirondack chair! Another good idea is to incorporate seating on or in walls or boulders that require climbing to reach. It's great to be king of the hill.

Designing with graded challenge is inclusive and productive. This kind of therapeutic garden might be conceived as a terrain park that offers a variety of self-directed movement and play opportunities. It is exercise in disguise, as play can be exercise. Incorporate hills and valleys, varying the slope from 30 percent to five percent, and high and low elements so children can bend, squat, and reach up high. Some engaging elements to include: herb planters hung on poles and fitted with pulleys to raise and lower them; a series of raised planting beds at varying heights; water pumps.

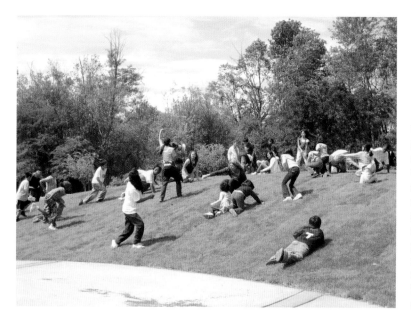

Children naturally gravitate to hills and mounds where they can climb up and roll, run, or slide down with complete abandon. A purposely designed hill would provide more level room at the bottom, which would stop the fun before children entered the path.

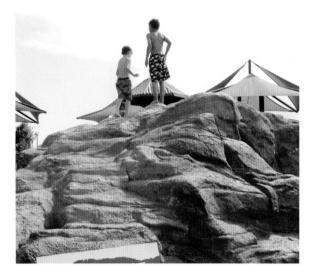

Manufactured stone is designed to simulate natural rock and can be included as a self-directed play element in a movement garden.

Child-friendly 24-inch-high railings can be used to do push-ups. A series of climbing elements like logs, tunnels constructed of bentwood or willow branches, suspension bridges, low balance beams, and stepping stones (spaced closer they are easier to traverse; further apart they become more difficult) offer tremendous movement and balance challenges for children. Incorporate a tree house accessed by steps, ramps, rope ladder, and pole—all different movement options, each with its own level of difficulty.

Wide paths aligned with universal design principles can curve or weave at sharp angles so children challenge themselves, constantly readjusting the way they use their bodies to walk, run, ride scooters, or bike. It takes more effort to successfully negotiate directional changes than to traverse a straight or curved line. Busier is better when designing therapeutic gardens to meet the needs of children with obesity.

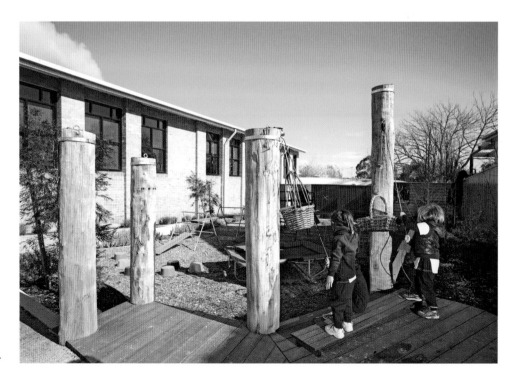

Another fun and creative exercise-in-disguise element: fit pillars with pulleys to raise and lower baskets to be filled and emptied.

Isabel Henderson Kindergarten

Isabel Henderson Kindergarten is located in Fitzroy, a suburb of Melbourne, Australia. Its outdoor play space, designed by Jeavons Landscape Architects (then Mary Jeavons Landscape Architects), provides a diverse environment for three- to five-year-olds, one designed to mitigate the increasingly sedentary and time-managed lives of children. The design incorporates existing features while simultaneously allowing the space to be multifunctional. Multipurpose spaces and adjustable, movable climbing elements encourage interactions with nature, complex socio-dramatic play, sensory/creative play, and physical activity. A seamless path enables all children to make their way through the garden. Sand pits that require separation from busy running and movement are protected by low plantings and other divisions within the space. A variety of natural (boulders, logs, raised beds) and man-made (fabric, sculpture by James Cattell) materials add sensory and tactile interest, define spaces, and provide distinctive character at a child-like scale. Water from rooftops collected in tanks sustainably provides for irrigation and water play. From intimate hidey holes and cubby spaces through to more open spaces for active play, the garden is a hub of activity for curious young children and staff to break the cycle of inactivity and instead to go outside—to play, explore, and grow.

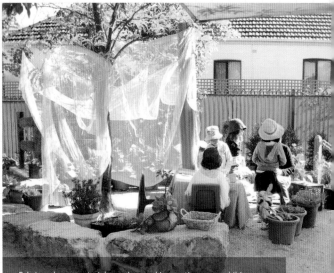

Fabric or loose materials can be used in creative ways; children sometimes fashion these materials into transitional nooks where they can chill out for the duration of play time or spend a few moments before moving on to larger, open spaces for active play.

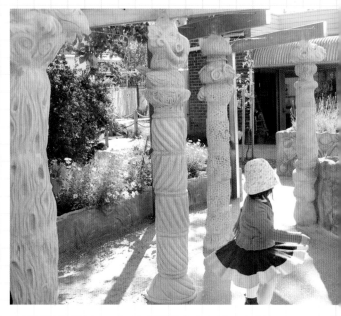

The design of the outdoor space empowers children to play as actively or quietly as they choose. Level pathways enable all children to move through with ease, to dance, twirl, or play a game of hide and seek.

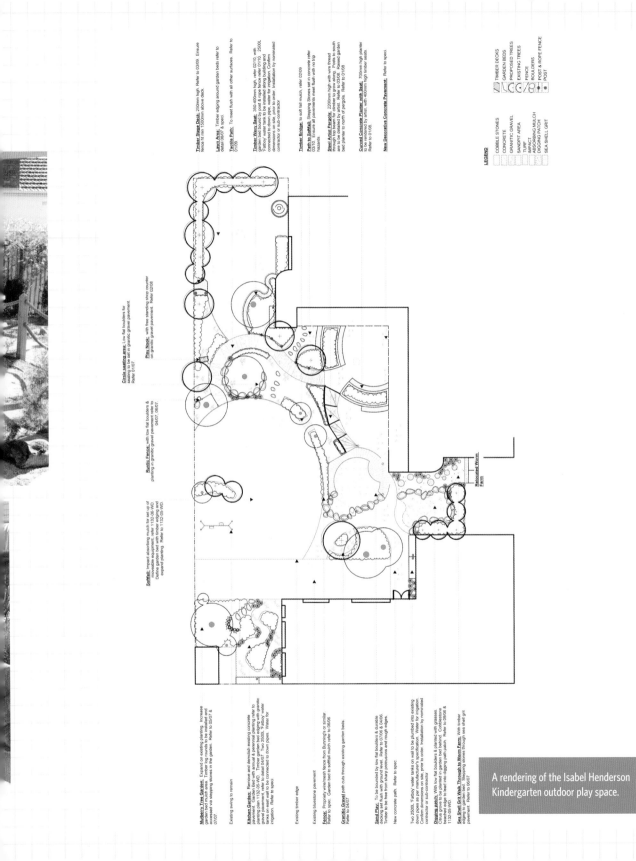

A rendering of the Isabel Henderson Kindergarten outdoor play space.

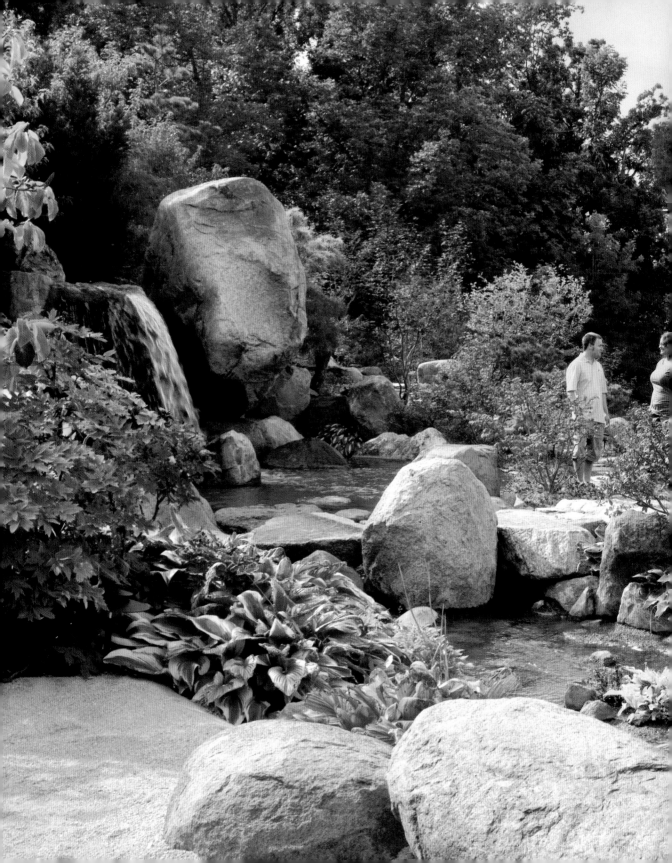

CHAPTER FOUR
GARDENS FOR SOLACE AND COMFORT

A garden for reflecting, remembering, and refuge offers profound solace and comfort to those experiencing loss, trauma, and displacement. Loss is fundamental to being human, and all will feel it at some point in their lives. Cemeteries and many public monuments are traditional models of places designed for remembrance, reflection, and healing. Designers will study such notable examples as the Vietnam War Memorial in Washington, D.C., and the Oklahoma City National Memorial. The impulse to create a place to mark a passing, express grief, ritually remember, and honor the dead is universal across cultures, ethnicities, and geographies. A place of remembrance is often an idealized version of nature; they can be visually powerful, whether modest or grand, from roadside shrines thick with flowers to 19th-century cemeteries conceived as botanic gardens. The beauty of trees and flowers is a counterpoint to death and a comfort to the grieving.

Honoring significant people and events, many memorial gardens are places of pilgrimage for collective remembrance. Visitors with broadly diverse outlooks are drawn to the Washington Mall's Vietnam Memorial by its enduring simplicity, accessibility, and stark beauty. Alongside the black granite memorial wall, inner and outer paths differ in width and material; the inner path allows people to linger at the wall to find the names of those lost, leave notes, and grieve without obstructing other visitors. The black stone reflects the viewer's image, linking it to the name of the missing loved one. The Vietnam Memorial was designed by artist and architect Maya Lin in 1982.

Shared by a developmental psychologist: In the span of less than two years, we lost my brother-in-law and mother-in-law. It was a really dark time in our lives—my husband felt lost, and I did, too. At the time, we lived close by a botanic garden in Georgia, and many mornings we found ourselves walking there, watching birds, looking at the clouds, and seeing the flora change with the seasons. It was an intensely quiet time for us; we seldom talked while in the garden, just held hands and strolled along the winding paths, remaining open to what would come next. After realizing that this morning walk through the garden was part of our healing process, a place for us to be quiet with our own thoughts, we decided to make a donation to the garden and have a bench dedicated in memory of my brother-in-law and mother-in-law. We got to choose the location. We selected a spot that was shady and looked out toward a pond, where at any given time, turtles and fish would swim lazily about, and gentle breezes rippled the water. We go to our bench every day. When I sit on our bench, I never fail to experience a deep connection with Jonah and Marge. It seems like they are with me. Remembering them in the garden has helped me deal with my grief. The bench has also become the place I go to when I have to think hard issues through and make decisions. It is a place I go to when I am happy and filled with joy. It is our special space.

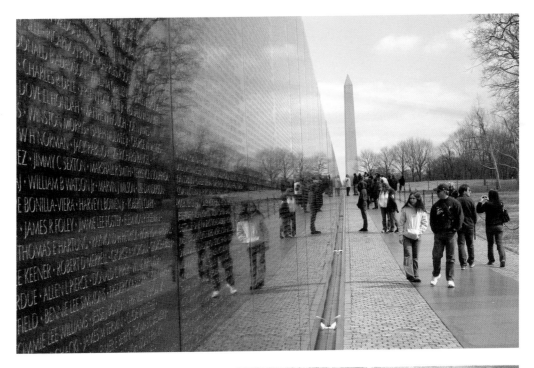

TOP At once intensely private and public, the Vietnam Memorial brings mourners and visitors together to reflect on the enduring effects of war. The path's design establishes two spaces: some can pause to reflect at the wall, and others can respectfully pass by.

BOTTOM Almost always a personal tribute and not designed by a professional, roadside memorials to loved ones are deeply meaningful to those who are grieving.

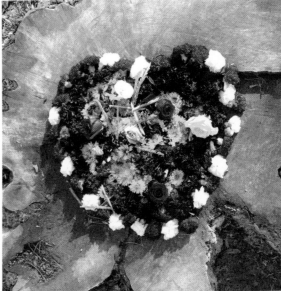

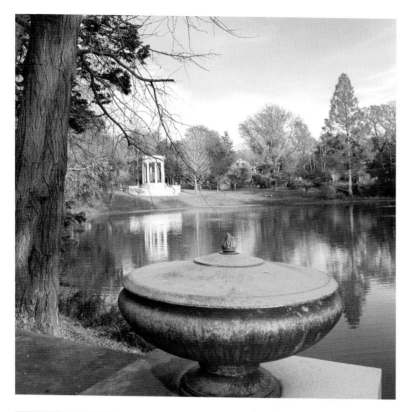

TOP Founded in 1831, Mount Auburn Cemetery in Massachusetts was conceived as both a cemetery and garden.

BOTTOM Landscape architecture firms can be called upon to renovate historically significant cemeteries such as the Ute Civil War Cemetery in Colorado.

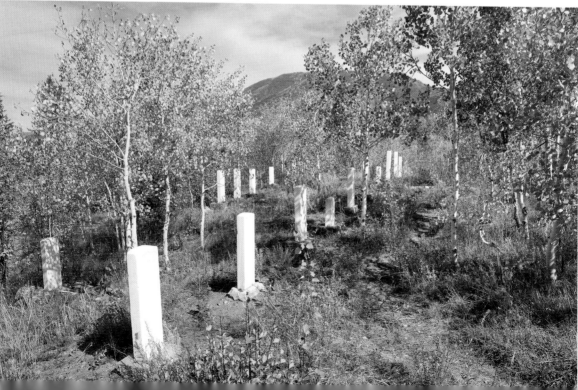

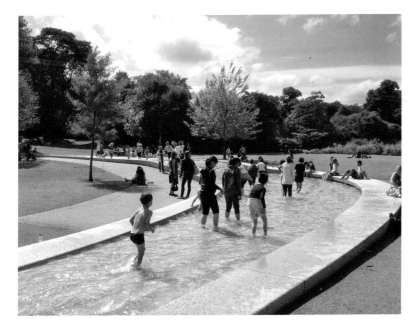

A lasting tribute to Lady Diana, her memorial brings people together in a spirit of joy—a fitting legacy.

A more recent example is a memorial garden that celebrates not just the loss but the life of Lady Diana Spencer. Her memorial in Hyde Park, London, designed by the landscape architectural firm of Gustafson Guthrie Nichol, centers on a water feature that is interactive and wheelchair-accessible. The water falls from a high point in two cascading granite runnels that join as they enter a calm pool, symbolizing different facets of Diana's life. On one side the water moves in a gentle, peaceful flow, and the other side is animated with falls, rills, and turbulence. Visitors are drawn to sit along the edge of the feature and run their fingers through the water. Water is the essential element that connects people with nature at the memorial. The vast open lawn surrounding the fountain welcomes picnicking and gathering, and every part of the garden accommodates all types of mobility.

The National AIDS Memorial Grove in San Francisco's Golden State Park is a serene and peaceful place to grieve and remember those taken by HIV/AIDS. Begun in 1988 at the height of the AIDS epidemic by a community devastated by the illness, it is a living memorial to all who were lost to it. Since 1991 volunteers have logged more than 60,000 hours, creating stone-paved gathering areas, placing benches and boulders, and planting native trees and shrubs. This restoration of the native ecology is both a real, tangible benefit and a metaphor that resonates with survivors as part of their healing process. For them and for all who remember, a forest canopy of redwoods and overhanging drifts of manzanita and other native shrubs are a consistent enveloping refuge in the garden's sequence of spaces.

Expanding on traditional memorial gardens and their innovations, gardens are now being designed to support healing for individuals and communities who are experiencing displacement and trauma. Displacement

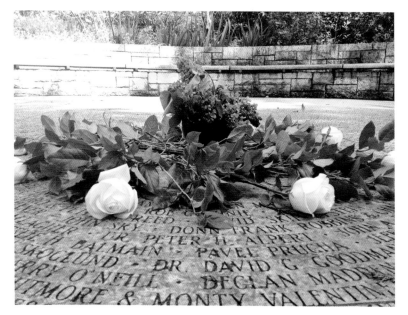

In the AIDS Memorial Grove, places for gathering and remembrance are fitted into the restored landscape, as here at the Circle of Friends.

is disruption from the familiar; trauma is experienced as deep distress that can be triggered by any kind of loss. This broader idea of loss includes not just the death of a loved one but loss of family relationships, home, health, and sense of self. Emotional and physiological responses to the deep wounds of displacement and trauma may include grief, pain, confusion, fear, and anxiety. These responses, if unmitigated, may lead to a sense of isolation, marginalization, and vulnerability. Such diverse groups as children and adults traumatized by horrific violence and war, refugees and immigrants, prisoners and the homeless, may find solace and comfort in a therapeutic garden, where, by being in and engaging with nature, they may safely experience brief or lasting release from the burdens they carry and that threaten to overtake their lives.

All the examples covered in this chapter are premised on the therapeutic benefits of nature interactions and the essential process of understanding user needs through participatory design to arrive at appropriate design solutions. Therapeutic gardens at healthcare facilities, correctional facilities, veterans hospitals, or homeless shelters have the capacity to support reflection and remembrance, and offer safe refuge to the most vulnerable. Reflection, remembrance, and refuge—these are the key themes of these gardens.

Gardens for Reflection, Remembrance, Refuge

Therapeutic gardens that support reflection, remembrance, and refuge incorporate a range of functional and emotive spaces, active and passive activities, and built sculptural elements to nurture and heal the mind and soul and foster a sense of coherence, connectivity, and resilience. Active engagement, the actual hands-on garden and maintenance work, may be a refuge to those who find physical work healing and cathartic. Engaging in music and other gentle and introspective rituals such as candle lighting, journaling, meditative walking, origami, reading, and observation may also be helpful to users.

REFLECTION

A garden that manifests pure reflection is the plaza at the Salk Institute in San Diego. Created by famed architect Louis Kahn, it features a simple stone water runnel and spillway. It is a memorial to time, solitude, light, and nature. Devoid of plants, it uses the natural biophilic elements of stone, water, and light to convey both powerful starkness and a sense of serenity. The water feature and plaza orientation extend and connect to a view of the Pacific Ocean, many miles away. The illusion of connection shrinks space and time, resulting in an enduring place. The plaza is a much-needed place for reflection, meditation, and dreaming, set apart from the routines and interruptions of the Salk's intense work environment. Such reflective interludes are found to refuel and reenergize an employee's return to concentration and creativity.

Gardens for reflection can be designed as quiet environments for health recovery, such as the Don Allen Memorial Garden and the Garden of Recovery, both designed by the Schmidt Design Group and located at San Diego's Sharp Mesa Vista Psychiatric Hospital. The Garden of Recovery is an essential component of inpatient and outpatient treatment programs for adolescents and adults. Half the garden includes active spaces for sports and play; the other half is a natural place to reflect, rethink, and recharge. These quiet components are essential to patients as they arrive and undergo treatment. Patients may be excessively withdrawn, prone to mood swings, and heavily medicated, with resulting

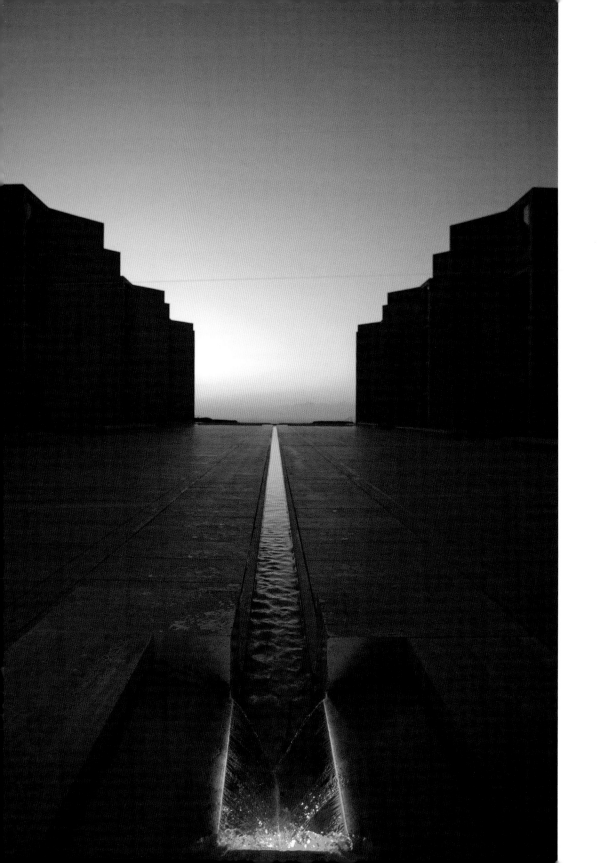

OPPOSITE Considered by many to be a masterpiece, the plaza at the Salk Institute for Biological Studies evokes a powerful sense of peace, serenity, and spaciousness.

disorientation, impaired balance, and coordination. In this state, they need a safe, peaceful, and solitary place for recovery, and also require close supervision. The garden is as immersively lush as it can be under these safety constraints. Beneath a light canopy of shade trees, essential in this sun-drenched climate, quiet sitting spaces are softly separated by ornamental grasses. A meandering sensory walk is framed by drifts of bright-flowering, low-growing perennials and textural succulents. The tenets of the hospital's recovery model—hope, connection, empowerment, self-responsibility, a meaningful life—are etched into the sidewalk. The Don Allen Memorial Garden is solely a place for reflection, prayer, and group therapy. Water is its most primal aspect. A waterfall muffles the sounds of conversation and is a visual focal point from a bridge that traverses a large koi pond. Together, the two gardens offer a range of active and quiet spaces to help those who struggle with mental illness or substance abuse experience greater control and choice in their recovery and ultimately find a sense of well-being.

Gardens for reflection can also be designed as spaces in which the focus is on therapeutic work and connection with others. Usually they will serve multiple purposes, with areas for reflection and spaces for

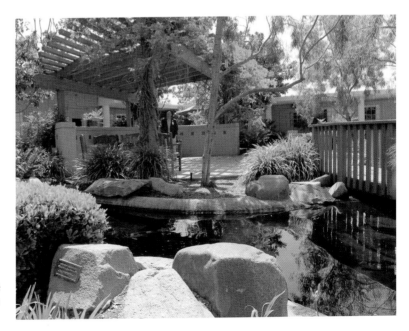

This shaded community space for group therapy and worship is used by patients at a drug and alcohol treatment center. A pond, especially one filled with koi and sited adjacent to seating areas for easy viewing, heightens the biophilic experience in a therapeutic garden.

programmed activities. The peace gardens of Bosnia and Herzegovina (BiH) demonstrate this duality, of both reflecting upon and working through traumatic memories. The first garden, the Stup Garden, was started in 1999 in Sarajevo, a city that endured a three-and-a-half-year siege in which 11,000 lost their lives and an additional 56,000 were wounded. As the Bosnian culture has few formal mechanisms for counseling or talk therapy, the garden plays a vital role. It grew out of a profound need for a place of reconciliation, where entrenched ethnic animosities might be peacefully confronted. Through the act of gardening, those who lost homes and loved ones could slowly return to a semblance of normality and regain a trust of their environment and their community. It is located on property given to the Bosnia Herzegovina Community Gardening Association by a survivor, who wanted to create a place for reconciliation on the site where her husband was killed.

Two-thirds of the garden consists of large plots for participants to grow food for themselves and for others in need. At the entry there is a communal greenhouse, a children's play area, a grove of fruit trees, and a small shaded gathering area with tables and seating. A pine tree marks the spot where the donor's husband was shot. Survivors cultivate food that was in short supply during and after the war. This purposeful activity distracts them from continually revisiting the horrors they have experienced; social connections with other gardeners are cultivated and stories emerge. Participants find solace and comfort in the common purpose and feel less burdened, isolated, and alone. In sharing the work of gardening, multiethnic survivors build collaboration, mutual trust, and friendship. The interethnic hatred that was propagated during the war is defused. In quiet, private moments in the renewed green space, gardeners reflect on the stark contrast it presents to the heavily bombed houses and buildings surrounding the site; they can recall a time when the city was vibrant, both with resplendent gardens and deep friendships across ethnicities. The gardens are seen as key to renewing the hope and trust that will construct a vision for the future.

Reflection takes on many meanings in the context of gardens and healing. It can be a time of meditation in the garden, a tuning in to the moment, a heightened awareness of the garden's colors, scents, and rhythms of sound which has the absorbing capacity to break a pattern of troubled thoughts. Reflection can be concentrated thinking through a situation, weighing options, and considering or making a difficult decision while

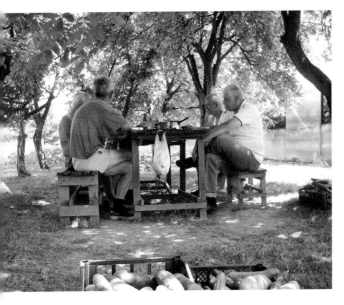

Previously estranged cross-ethnic relationships can be healed and mediated in a garden's spirit of fellowship and renewal.

gently stroking the silky leaves of silver sage (*Salvia argentea*) or slowly walking the paths of a labyrinth. For one parent whose child was very ill, the Stenzel Garden at Good Samaritan Hospital in Portland, Oregon, was the place she came to pray for her critically ill child.

Reflection can be privately confronting denial and loss and accepting a new reality or challenge. It can also be an emptying of the mind or exiting an existing routine to make way for alternative ways of thinking, opening up the possibility of creative ideas and decision-making. The therapeutic garden that provides gentle interactions with nature offers users experiencing distress opportunity for reflection and as such engages or renews the body, the senses, and the mind. Distant views in nature of mountains, sky, and water allow the mind to wander and be introspective. In a garden of reflection, this depth of field is structured by massing elements in multiple planes. The eye and mind are free to travel through foreground, middle, and background spaces.

Focal points are used for meditation, using any or all senses. The movement and sound of water mesmerizes. In winter, the form and texture of a tree with sculptural branching and peeling bark captures the eye. A

Depth of field leads the eye out into the garden and allows visitors to escape into the landscape. The balance of foreground, middle ground, and far ground can be constructed through plants and architectural features.

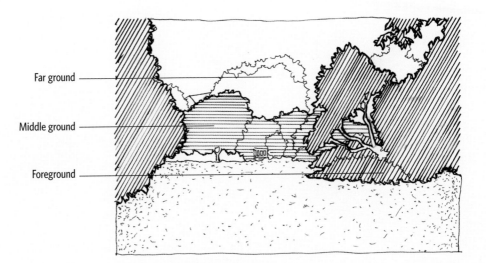

Far ground

Middle ground

Foreground

background that contrasts and recedes distinguishes the focal point. A variety of comfortable chairs and benches and windows for looking out into the garden can be oriented to a vista or focal point, gently redirecting users away from their burdens.

REMEMBRANCE

The Remembrance Garden in Hampstead, London, a part of Freedom from Torture's Natural Growth Project, was created by and for a refugee community—victims of torture from around the world. Its series of planted beds with specific purposes—peace, healing, vegetable, children's, rose gardens—are accessed through concrete and stepping stone paths and swaths of open lawn. In addition to the garden beds, there is a greenhouse, pond, summerhouse, shed, and gathering patio. Clients come to the gardens with tremendous emotional and physical scars. They are tormented by the past, fear the present, and question what, if any, future awaits them. Many have difficulty relating to other people and are consumed by fear and anger; they find it easier and safer to engage with nature—to talk to a bird, smell a flower, caress a leaf, plant an herb—than to interact with people.

The goal of the Natural Growth Project is that clients learn to associate these positive experiences in the garden with optimism for the present. In

Damaged or broken from the trauma and atrocities they have suffered, clients come to the Natural Growth Project's Remembrance Garden to heal and become whole again.

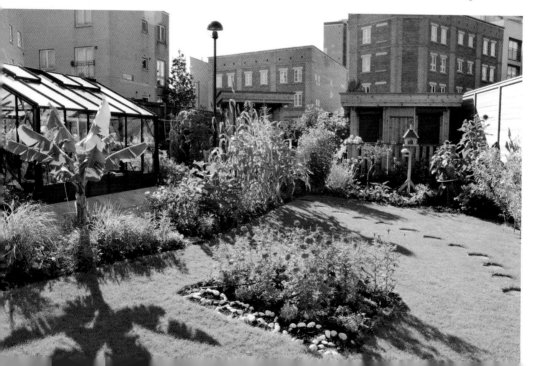

time these positive memories may replace or diminish the horrors of the past, allowing clients to feel safe and to trust themselves and others once more. Many of the garden elements were imagined and created by the clients to remind them of home. The community wood-fired bread oven in the Remembrance Garden is a unifying, iconic place for these clients from diverse cultures to come together around the common activity of bread making. While mixing and baking the dough, the participants often talk effortlessly about their lives, sharing stories and recalling the past.

One woman, who wished to grow plants she knew to be healing, resurrected what had once been a vegetable and herb garden. At the center she created a heart-shaped planting of heartsease (*Viola tricolor*), representing heartache and longing. Other clients began participating and caring for the garden, and many now come to harvest the medicinal and culinary herbs, whose scents and flavors trigger immediate memories of home. Other gardens within the Remembrance Garden reference childhood gardens—for example, the small rose garden planted by a client who rediscovered the scents and beauty of the roses she raised in her country of origin.

Through involvement in the gardens of the Natural Growth Project, clients acclimate to their new home in England. The clients discover new plants reminiscent of home and also cultivate seeds given to them by relatives and friends. The garden links memories of home with the reality of a new climate, soils, and cultural preferences. A bridge is created that links the best of the past with a positive new start. It is a place where both plants and memories are cultivated and renewed. Clients are encouraged to be expressive, to create plantings, murals, art work, and spaces that bring their past to the present. A program of talk therapy in the garden helps clients come to terms with the deeply traumatic events that threaten to shatter their lives. The garden is an accepting place where memories of these events can be acknowledged and confronted. Therapists use metaphors related to nature and the garden to bring to mind and illuminate the struggles their clients face. Good memories are savored as touchstones.

Reconnecting to memories elicits conflicting interpretations and complex emotions. For some, it may be valuable to recall painful memories, to acknowledge and confront them in a process of recovery and reconciliation. A garden designed to provide comfortable, calm, and quiet places with evocative scents, sounds, and colors can bring its user to a more peaceful frame of mind. Places to sit (alone or together), elements to observe, and active spaces at which to interact with the garden at differing levels of participation will enhance the meaning of a garden for remembrance. The participatory design process is always critical but is especially so in such a garden; it is vital to learn about and take into account the intensely personal past memories of a community and its individuals.

Memorialization is an important act of remembrance for survivors, whether in the form of a garden as a whole, designed to evoke the spirit of place connected to a particular person or group, or as a small marker within the garden to remember specific people or events. These markers may be favorite plants or inscriptions of names, narration, or poetry on bricks, stone, or metal. Memorial gardens invite rituals of honoring and celebration using shrines, lighted candles, bells, and other centering elements.

Among the early gardens created specifically as a memorial garden in a healthcare facility is a set of three gardens completed in 1999 at Rady Children's Hospital San Diego. They honor the memory of Carley, who died of

Crossing a bridge is a metaphor for passage, to a new place and a fresh beginning. Bridges are the present that connects the past to the future.

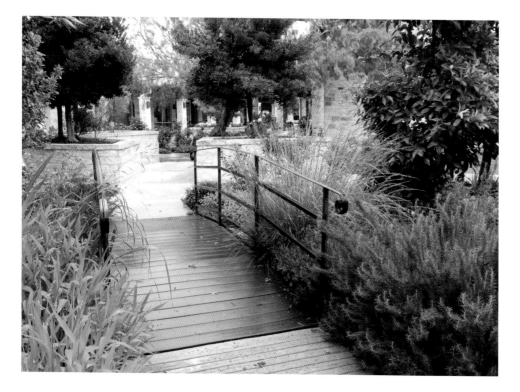

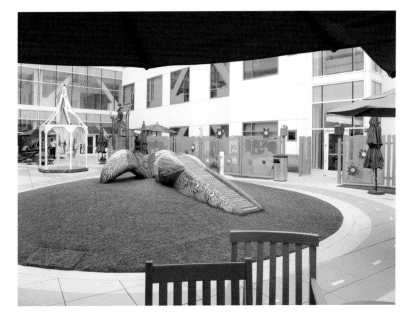

While there is no living plant material in Carley's Magical Garden, it is still highly engaging; children happily play in the garden or view it from their hospital windows.

leukemia in 1997. The gardens were inspired by her imagination and curiosity about the spiders, insects, and birds she observed on the grounds while being treated at the hospital. All three, the Garden of Dreams, the Buggy Garden, and the Friendship Garden, feature ceramic mosaic and bronze sculptures of animals that children can climb on and interact with. The animals are comical, and humor and playfulness, particularly in the hospital context, releases stress for children and their families. The gardens, initiated by her parents, express Carley's vibrant character and provide other children undergoing treatment with colorful spaces to look into while confined to their hospital rooms. Carley's Magical Garden, recently installed on a second-floor terrace, contains no living plants—a response to a need to reduce the risk of infection from germs and mold. Despite the lack of nature, the new garden contains many engaging features for children, among them a playhouse, a treasure hunt for 12 golden goose eggs, and a century-old boat, which invites young patients to climb aboard and set sail on imaginary adventures.

Memorial gardens are also found in religious facilities, university campuses, and public parks, buildings, and plazas. Following the tragic Oklahoma City bombing of 1995, an extensive remembrance memorial was erected on the site of the attack. In one of its many metaphorical touches, an American elm that took the brunt of the blast and endured is now the focal point of a newly planted grid of fruit and nut trees; the survivor tree represents resilience, and the orchard honors the many rescuers who came to assist the injured. Gardens of remembrance and memorialization aligning with therapeutic programs (such as Carley's gardens) and individual or collective rituals (as seen in Oklahoma City) help people find healing connections within themselves and with their community.

REFUGE

One of the earliest gardens of refuge created for people with HIV/AIDS is the Joel Schnaper Memorial Garden at New York's Terence Cardinal Cooke Health Care Center. In its original form and constructed entirely with donations and volunteer labor, the 3,000-square-foot rooftop garden was dedicated to Joel Schnaper, a landscape architect specializing in urban gardens who died of AIDS. At the time of the original design in 1994, the illness was terminal, much was uncertain about its progression, and all touched by the disease felt vulnerable to the assault of its myriad disabling conditions. As landscape architect David Kamp later recalled, "That uncertainty led to a design that employed simple basic principles of flexibility, opportunity, and choice. Those principles have served the garden well over the years" (Rainey 2010). Kamp had a direct and continual dialogue with the center's physicians, therapists, and nurses throughout the original design process.

Then and today, the garden is located adjacent to the AIDS unit, which serves 156 residents. Five green rooms provide comfort and access to nature with an abundant variety of textural plantings including birches, wisteria, and large-leafed annuals. The flexible use of planters and trellises with screening vines gives both patients viewing the garden from their rooms and people outside in the garden the varying amounts of privacy needed to feel safe. Choice is also provided by movable cushioned furniture, allowing patients and caregivers to create their own retreats to be together. Planters are installed at waist height so that the sensory-rich experience of gardening is available to all users. Patients grow herbs, fruits, and vegetables; therapeutic horticulture activities feel like working in the garden at home. There are active spaces for yoga and

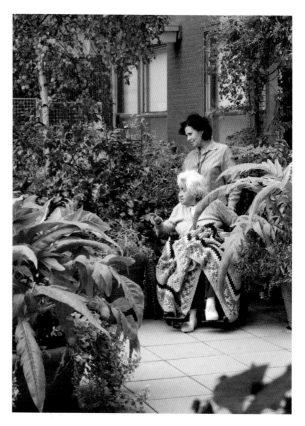

Wheelchair and standing-height planters increase the usability and experience of the garden for patients.

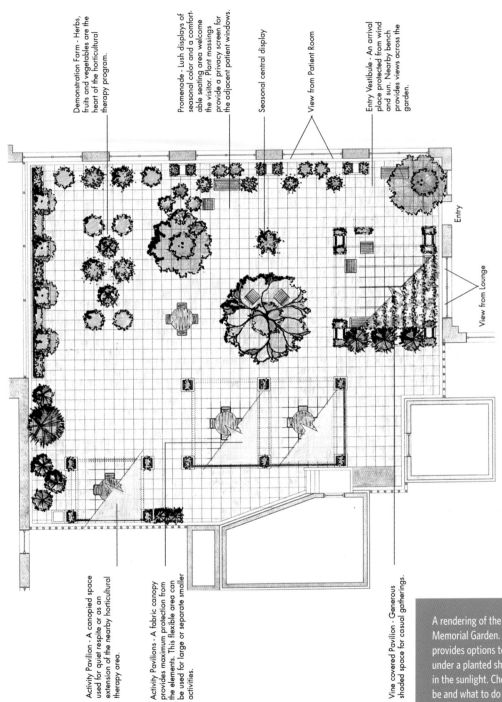

Demonstration Farm - Herbs, fruits and vegetables are the heart of the horticultural therapy program.

Promenade - Lush displays of seasonal color and a comfortable seating area welcome the visitor. Plant massings provide a privacy screen for the adjacent patient windows.

Seasonal central display

View from Patient Room

Entry Vestibule - An arrival place protected from wind and sun. Nearby bench provides views across the garden.

Entry

View from Lounge

Activity Pavilion - A canopied space used for quiet respite or as an extension of the nearby horticultural therapy area.

Activity Pavilions - A fabric canopy provides maximum protection from the elements. This flexible area can be used for large or separate smaller activities.

Vine covered Pavilion - Generous shaded space for casual gatherings.

A rendering of the Joel Schnaper Memorial Garden. The garden provides options to all visitors to sit under a planted shade structure or in the sunlight. Choice of where to be and what to do is a particularly powerful experience for patients.

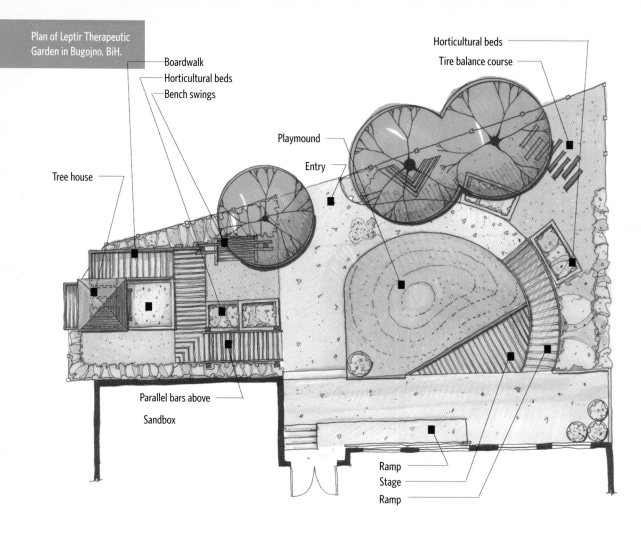

Plan of Leptir Therapeutic Garden in Bugojno, BiH.

Boardwalk
Horticultural beds
Bench swings

Horticultural beds
Tire balance course

Playmound

Entry

Tree house

Parallel bars above

Sandbox

Ramp
Stage
Ramp

other group activities and quiet niches for contemplation or visiting with a friend. There are varied exposures to the elements, and several shade structures minimize contact with the sun, as medications for those with HIV/AIDS increase photosensitivity. Many design strategies are directed to those with mobility impairments. Low-glare concrete-textured pavers and automatic door openers allow patients to use the garden independently. Wide walkways accommodate wheelchairs, and walkers and ramps are gently sloped.

In 2005, building upgrades necessitated that the garden be rebuilt using more suitable and sustainable materials. The renovation coincided with a broader concept for the garden to serve not only individuals with HIV/AIDS but the facility's larger community of long-term-care patients and residents. While continuing to support the concept of refuge, new and enhanced features intended to meet the needs of a more varied patient population, such as a musical performance area and additional pavilions for active or passive activities, were added.

In Bosnia and Herzegovina, disabled children face severe discrimination and prejudice. The Leptir Therapeutic Garden for children with disabilities (and their families) serves as a refuge from a culture that stigmatizes them. The garden is located in Bugojno, near the center of town, where its visibility to the community helps the children gain acceptance. The garden nurtures each user through a range of nature interactions to support all aspects of their development—social, psychological, physical, sensory, and cognitive. The sensorial gardens offer smell, touch, and sight experiences to help focus and improve attention. The climbing trees, jumping stones, and rolling hills encourage physical exploration and interaction with nature. These are new opportunities for the children who have neither natural areas to play in nor accessible play equipment. In this garden, the two are woven together. Cognitive skills are honed through sensory and movement experiences. The children and their families find playful escape and a safe refuge within the garden. The stigma of being differently-abled is abated. In the garden, children can strive, fail, and succeed without judgment or disapproval.

Finding refuge in a therapeutic garden is finding a place of comfort and safety. In an institutional setting, this haven might be the only escape from the monotony of routines. For some, refuge is found in familiar associations such as to a remembered or idealized home, as in the Schnaper garden. For others it is an escape, a place that is novel and stimulates curiosity, as in the Leptir garden. Both gardens represent a new beginning. Safety and a high level of accessibility supports refuge. For those whose lives have been shaped by threats, prejudice, and abuse, a place free of these burdens provides relief from stress, a place to recover, to reconnect with themselves or with others, to build resilience, and find acceptance.

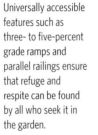

Universally accessible features such as three- to five-percent grade ramps and parallel railings ensure that refuge and respite can be found by all who seek it in the garden.

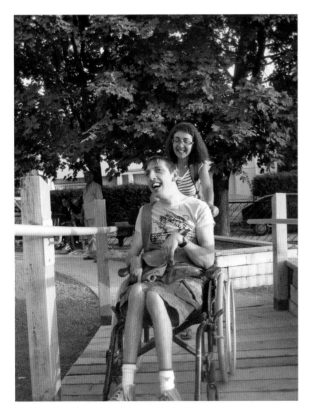

CLOSER LOOK

Rosecrance

Located on 50 scenic acres in Rockford, Illinois, the Rosecrance Griffin Williamson Campus is an innovative 80-bed adolescent substance abuse treatment facility, a place where patients arrive to reflect on a more positive way forward. The garden was designed by Kurisu International under the direction of Hoichi Kurisu. Nestled within a backdrop of thick woodland, the garden not only inspires reflection but is a refuge from the tribulations associated with substance abuse, whether directly as a patient or as one who has come to support their loved one. Mature trees and an abundance of other sensory-rich plantings invite patients and guests to become engaged with and immersed in healing nature. Being outdoors, hearing the rush of water, the feel of the

Large boulders serve multiple purposes in the design: they function as seating, they define space, and they serve as bridges and walkways.

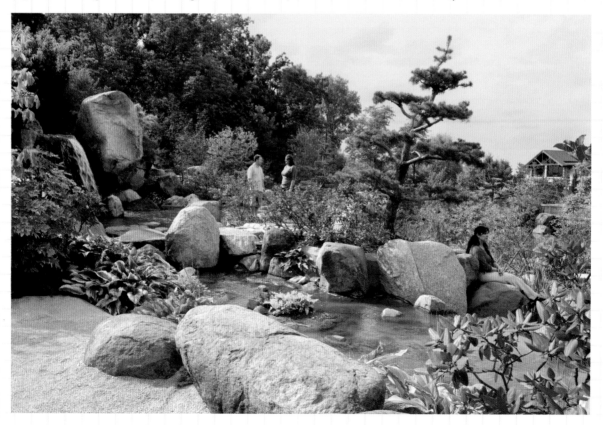

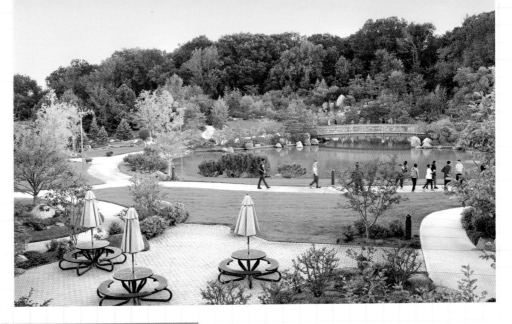

Well-maintained and level paths increase the likelihood that teens will be drawn to use them. Research finds that walking in nature decreases depressive symptoms.

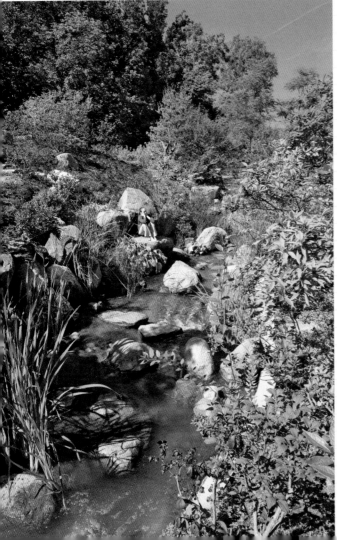

breeze, taking in the views within and beyond the garden that provide soft fascination—all help to foster relaxation and focus. Water represents the life blood; reflective water elements include a koi pond and falls, which cascade over large rocks in a pattern of 12 steps, symbolizing the recovery process. The experimental therapies staff works with patients to use the garden, when weather permits, for meditation, sensory enrichment, horticultural therapy, and journaling. Serenity circles are designed as places for families to gather with their loved one, and as refuges for patients, who use them as places to read, draw, remember, or reflect in a safe and nurturing environment.

Biophilic elements— plants, stone, and water—help facilitate a connection, or reconnection, between self and the greater world.

Gardens for Healthcare Facilities

Therapeutic gardens that nurture reflection and remembrance hold the utmost value to patients and to caring family members, friends, and staff in the realm of healthcare. Those who are sick need someplace to go that relieves the stresses they deal with each day of their treatment. One nurse talked of 12-hour operating-room shifts that required long periods of focus. For her, just viewing the garden in passing is replenishment. Whether the garden is embraced or viewed through a window, these green sanctuaries are reminders of the vitality of natural systems when life seems fragile.

The most sensitive way to design contemplation spaces is to create rooms within the garden or throughout the hospital complex. Green options include niche spaces defined by living walls, as by espaliered trees

A quiet garden nook offers users solace and comfort. It is a much-needed place to visit with friends, to take stock, and to make decisions about themselves or loved ones.

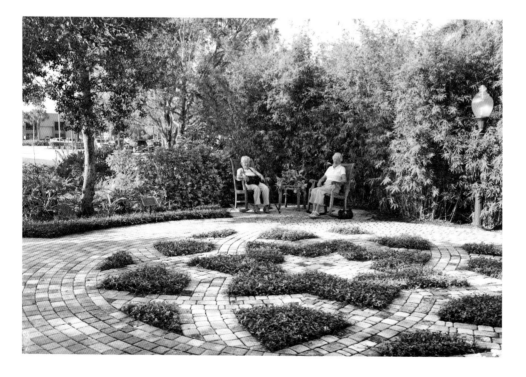

or vines trained up mesh fencing. The strategy is to build spaces that feel private and intimate, and which are readily understood as welcoming. They are best located close to garden entries, for access to those with mobility impairments, but set apart from main paths, both for privacy and the sense of getting away. Multiple retreats provide users with choices and allow them to find, at a particular moment of need, a place in the garden to meditate and center themselves, or to consider and process all that may be happening. In the best examples, a garden's forms and elements guide users to find and explore the reflective spaces. Users may not be conscious of how much they need these quiet escapes nestled within the therapeutic garden until they find themselves embraced by them.

In Japan's first therapeutic garden, designed by Yoshisuke Miyake of SEN, Inc., and installed in 2004 at the Kansai Rosai Hospital, one of the garden's nine "rooms," the Garden of Memories, is accessible only with a key; its white flowers, lightly scented plants, and small water feature create a quiet and tranquil for families in need of a more private space to grieve, to remember, and to reflect. At the Jacqueline Fiske Garden of Hope in Jupiter, Florida, a graceful stand of bamboos forms a semi-transparent screen around a small seating area set just off the main hub of the courtyard garden; the space is often used for family meetings and quiet contemplation.

Cancer Lifeline in Seattle supports those diagnosed with cancer and their families. Among the three rooftop therapeutic gardens at the center, the smallest space is a grieving room. The seating is arranged out of view of hallway windows. A trellis vined with akebia subtly screens the seating to reveal its availability to potential users before they intrude on an occupant's private moments. At the center of the grief room are three copper and glass sculptures, where users may light a candle or leave a note or object in memory of a loved one. Under the sculpture is a small water fountain composed of black river rocks overlaid with mosses.

DESIGN CONSIDERATIONS

Every strategy of the design can aim to amplify softness, quietude, and the garden's gentle, graceful, and verdant aspects. The language of escape can be incorporated into the garden by paths that gently curve and meander. There are strategies to mask the ambient and obtrusive noises that prevail in healthcare facilities. Sounds include compressor pumps, heating and cooling tower noises, buzzers, alarms, and announcement systems;

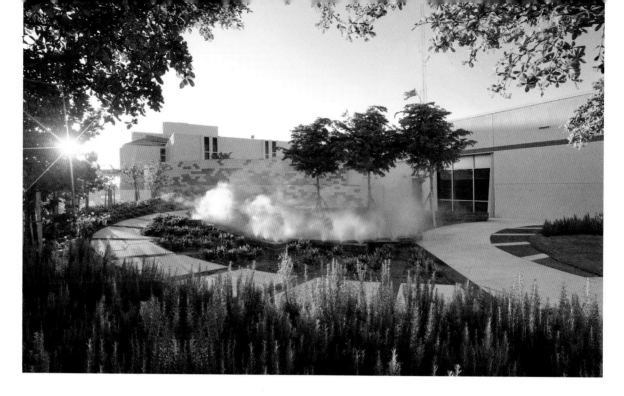

effective strategies to mask them include falling water, rustling bamboo, wind chimes, and green screens and hedges. Simple amenities such as seat cushions, heaters, and misters bring an extra dimension of care and compassion to the garden. In hotter climates, vertically oriented misters can serve as walls.

Memorial plants, tributes to those who have walked this path before, can be woven into planting areas. In some gardens, such plants have a modest plaque, but in other gardens they are anonymous, known only to the donors and their extended community. Names to be remembered can be inscribed on glass leaves adorning a sculptural tree, as seen in the Les and Betty Krueger Family Healing Garden on the rooftop of the Harrison Medical Center in Bremerton, Washington.

Many people wish to be memorialized at healthcare facilities, or for that matter, any other donor-funded garden project. Often a generous donor, a beloved family member, or prominent civic leader has stipulated that part of their estate is to be donated to a healthcare facility after their passing. A therapeutic garden is especially effective at creating a living testament to whoever is being remembered.

TOP Another material to consider when designing rooms in a garden: misters are alternatives to green or manufactured walls.

BOTTOM There are many innovative ways to honor donors who choose to be identified. Glass leaves on this sculptural tree are etched with donor names.

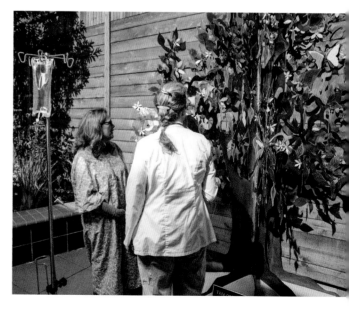

Gardens for Private Residences

Residential therapeutic gardens might be designed as a memorial for a loved one who has passed or to honor someone who has overcome a major life obstacle. They are highly individualized gardens, compelling in that they memorialize or honor someone in a most intimate place: home. The garden can be used or viewed on a daily basis, throughout the seasons. While donor gardens at healthcare or other venues are equated with some degree of ownership by virtue of a personal and financial commitment, a therapeutic garden at a private residence belongs solely to the homeowner.

Designers are rarely asked by clients to design and install this type of a home therapeutic garden, but there is a notable example to consider.

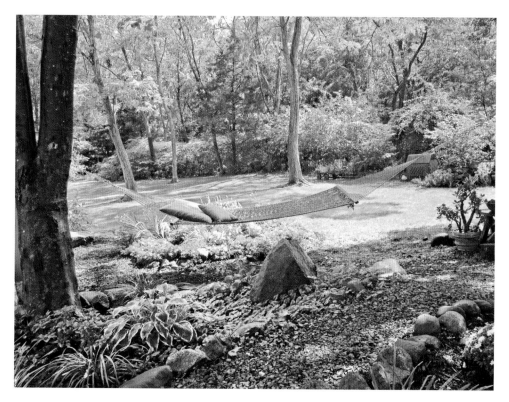

For people recovering from illness, places to rest like hammocks and lounge chairs greatly enhance a garden's tranquility and comfort.

Hope in Bloom is an organization in the Boston area that designs and installs therapeutic gardens at the homes of people who have survived breast cancer. Each garden is designed to meet the specific needs and desires of the client, and accordingly each is different in scale, size, and features. One Hope in Bloom client proclaimed her new garden as her favorite place on the planet, full of delight, enchantment, bliss, and peace, the place where she, as a survivor of cancer, goes to reflect on the joys and blessings in her life. A majestic tree provides ample shade, and under its canopy are multiple places to sit and gaze at the plantings and distinctive pieces of art appearing in every nook of the garden. There is a gently curved pathway to walk along and a comfortable hammock for reading or resting. An avid gardener herself, the client helped with the design and continues to contribute to this work in perpetual progress.

DESIGN CONSIDERATIONS

Intensely individualized, therapeutic gardens designed for homeowners may be installed in back or front yards, on a condominium balcony or terrace, or even as an indoor living sanctuary. What does the client want the garden to represent: memories about a loved one who has died, courage and survival, or a refuge from daily life? For example, consider how the loved one's hobbies or passions can be reflected in the garden; an avid bird watcher may be memorialized with plantings that attract birds—graceful bird feeders, a birdbath, and a cozy bench with a side table where a pair of binoculars and birder guide can be at the ready. A terrace or balcony garden needs to be skillfully designed to balance the public, shared-living element with privacy. While keeping with association rules, a first step is to screen the perimeter of the balcony so that the interior space can be a serene and private haven to remember a beloved family member, friend, or pet. Clever use of small-scale furniture and plantings will be important to ensure that the space does not end up feeling cluttered and claustrophobic. Indoor gardens with an arrangement of plants or a living wall may also serve a client well. Home therapeutic gardens inherently foster ownership, but they still benefit from a participatory design process. Work with clients so that the design includes and accommodates personally meaningful ritual elements, such as candles, a journaling desk, drums, chimes, sculpture, or a small water feature.

Gardens for Underserved and Marginalized Populations

Many underserved and marginalized user groups—children, inmates, refugees, homeless, veterans—experience the trauma of disconnection. These groups are united by a sense of displacement from community, family, and friends, which often results in loss of identity, well-being, and sense of place. The process of creating nurturing outdoor environments that provide people, both young and old, with opportunities to process

Involving a community in the design process demonstrates a high level of commitment to understanding and respecting their needs. When language barriers present, using icons and photos to illustrate concepts is useful.

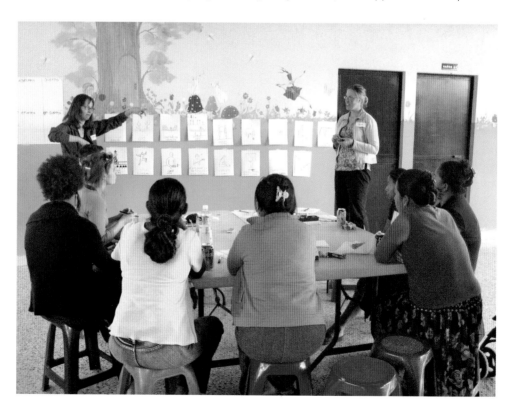

their losses and rebuild attachments to others and to place requires research and dialogue to understand these communities and to learn their individual stories. Victims of trauma can manifest significant physical and psychological symptoms, including being more susceptible to illness and slow to recover. Some experience a downward spiral of depression or other mental health issues, commit violent acts, or are filled with despair. In accordance with the biophilia hypothesis, discussed earlier, the inherent properties of nature in therapeutic gardens have the greatest benefit for those most disconnected and distressed.

As with any garden created for a specific vulnerable user group, gardens for marginalized populations need to be designed with the utmost degree of sensitivity to, compassion for, and understanding of the people who will be using them. They must respond to and reflect the values, cultural background, and identity the end users bring with them. Therapeutic gardens—active, passive, or a combination of both—have the potential to help underserved and marginalized users groups reflect on and reconnect with themselves, their community, and cultural identities. Working closely through a participatory design process with the user groups and community advocates is important. It builds community and consensus and creates a sense of pride in and ownership of a space that feels like home.

As awareness of the multifaceted benefits of therapeutic gardens increases, their relevance to underserved populations is beginning to be recognized and duly acknowledged. Post-occupancy studies of all projects should be undertaken to validate their importance as a mechanism for healing. Successful projects are the precedents for future design innovations.

Gardens for Marginalized Children

Like all children, children who live at the margins of society have little to no control over the conditions of their home environment. In Guatemala, too many children are vulnerable to a cycle of poverty and constant exposure to multiple traumatic experiences: war, violence, sexual and physical abuse, lack of education, poor diets, and toxic exposure; and in urban areas, refugee and homeless families have little experience of nature. Many NGOs are helping with programs to support health and education; one, Safe Passage, responded to the nature deficit by building a play garden park around its educational facilities. The Children's Garden of Hope in Guatemala City serves the families who live in shanties adjacent to the garbage dump and integrates the NGO's educational and social support activities throughout the extensive garden spaces. The walled garden is a safe place, giving children daily access to nature play and opportunities to lessen the effects of mood swings, depression, hyperactivity, and attention deficit disorder. The core of the design is the linkages between

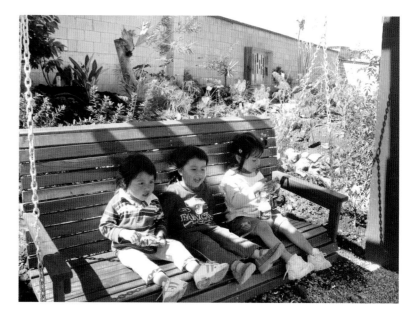

A bench swing offers varied therapeutic benefits—a place to gather, to talk, and to seek comfort from others.

active and passive play activities through a network of spaces; these differ in style, character, and therapeutic objectives, offering a range of experiences from formal to wild, tactile, aromatic, colorful, and humorous. On an exploratory path are hanging musical instruments made from found metal objects with tethered bamboo mallets to use for striking and working out feelings of anger—or simply to create music. The choice of spaces and activities enables children either on their own or encouraged by a care provider to seek the most appropriate place to meet their needs.

In the community design process, parents and children who would be using the Garden of Hope asked for plants whose colors and scents would attract insects and birds and remind them of their rural homes. The arbors are enveloped with sweet-scented vines. Children use the bench swings under the arbors in one area as a source of comfort. The gentle rocking motion, the quiet shaded space, and sense of enclosure are appealing to children feeling stressed, socially challenged, or seeking a calming break from intense activities. Each swing is large enough to accommodate several children with a caregiver. Sometimes children sit passively on the swing and observe children engaged in activities within the garden. They snuggle, snack, listen to a storyteller, and socialize.

Children and their families also use the bench swing as a place to come together when grieving for a lost family member. Tragically, many young adults in Guatemala are victims of escalating gang violence. Creating modest sanctuaries within the garden offers comfort to those who need to express their grief, whether alone or together with a family member. Children in a raw state of confusion and pain may not be in control of their emotions, so offering a range of spaces will accommodate all stages of the grieving process. At some point children will ask questions, as death may be mysterious and incomprehensible to them. Including a place for a family to gather and talk, such as a bench swing or other intimate space, will support their need when that occasion arises.

A counterpoint to the passive and contemplative experiences unfolds in the active play areas of the

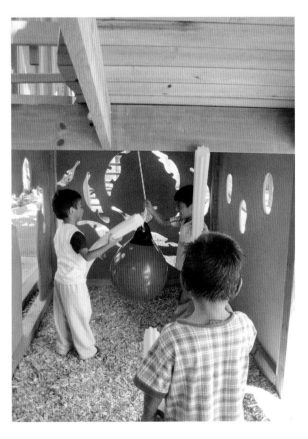

Elements such as suspended punching bags or balls to bat provide scaffolding for children to act out aggression and anger.

garden, which feature bridges, climbing structures, climbing mounds, tree houses, and slides. Through pretend play and physical exploration, the children escape from memories that trigger anxiety and sadness and engage in more improvisational and carefree social exchanges with their siblings and peers.

A walk through a bentwood tunnel flanked with fuzzy-topped grasses provides an abundance of positive distraction, wonder, and mystery.

DESIGN CONSIDERATIONS

It is important for designers to understand the impacts of loss and trauma on children, that they can be profound and have lasting effects. The erosion of safe, reliable, coherent social structures can come from homelessness, natural disaster, isolating illness, abuse, and consequences of war. Children's physical development may be stunted; they may demonstrate learning and attentional problems, be disruptive and aggressive at home or in school, or retreat far into themselves. Many studies of child health have shown the positive global impact of nature on many aspects of development. For children with emotional and social challenges, helping to care for and cultivate a garden offers a distraction from memories of pain and loss. A study of over 300 typically developing children found that access to nearby nature had a buffering effect on stress and adversity, which improved their sense of resilience, mastery, and self-worth (Wells and Evans 2003). In a safe, natural environment children can feel free to explore. Stress is reduced as they engage in activities that hone fine and gross motor skill development, improve social interactions, and boost self-esteem. Green spaces offer many benefits for children including play, education, nutrition, and skill-building for future vocations.

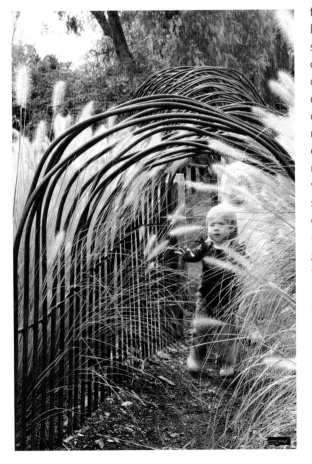

Play is an integral part of childhood. Typically, children use play as a way to investigate their environment, socialize, and move. For children who can, unscripted, self-directed play promotes healthy self-image as children are free to engage in or to observe others in pretend play, and learn about the physical world beyond themselves as they manipulate objects and move. Given the opportunity to direct their outdoor

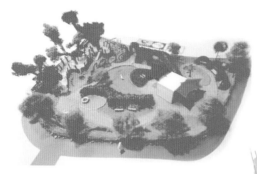

Apple Core Space

The patterned metal entrance gate and living willow tunnel provide a multi-sensory experience, taking the user out of the hospital setting and into the secure play space.
The central wet pour area, sheltered by the play house canopies creates a safe flexible space for educational, performance or free mobile play, with balls, bikes, mats and other materials stored conveniently near in the play house. The central surface is patterned with a maze to encourage focus and mobility.
The surrounding grass amphitheatre bank can be used for sitting & observing, rolling & tumbling & climbing.
The adjacent self binding gravel surfaced willow tunnels allow exploration, hide & seek & den play. The multisensory qualities of the willow and the surfaces of the Apple core area give full opportunities for mobility, tactile, auditory & visual healing play. Sculpture seating provides scope for intimate seating and observation.

Tree Houses Space

An exciting, inclusively accessible network of aerial walkways, platforms & tree houses created around the framework and beneath the sheltering canopies of the existing oak & beech trees.
From this structure a range of attached swings, slides, ladders, canopies & ground level set trampoline give a huge range of challenges and mobility exercise options for children of all abilities and their carers.
The ground surfaceof reinforced turf, self binding gravel & wet pour to retain the natural woodland feel.
The adjacent existing boundary hedgebank will be refurbished, fitted with a timber pale and trellis fence planted with woodland plants to enrich the spaces natural sensory value.
Tree house dens and sculpture seating provides scope for intimate seating and observation, protected behind a linear, willow screen planted mound.

17   Scramble net with log stepping stone access
18   Grass rolling bank (mesh reinforced)
19   Living willow & hazel poles low hoopped fence
20   Wooden carved animals & balance beams
21   Carved log seats & stools
22   Trampoline (ground inset)
23   Nest swing (bi-directional)
24   Inclusive use swing (bi-directional)
25   Wet pour surface
26   Mesh reinforced turf surface
27   Self binding gravel surface
28   Timber deck rollway/ walkway & timber pale ballustrade
29   Timber deck platform, landings & timber pale ballustrade
30   Musical / tactile / visual play elements on ballustrade
31   Tensile deck canopy (anti-climb) fixed around existing tree stem
32   Timber pale gate
33   Log seating beneath lower platform
34   Den beneath upper platform
35   Inclusive double slide & access platform
36   Access ladder
37   Refurbished existing hedgebank with timber pale fence & trellis
38   New section of stone faced hedgebank timber pale fence & trellis
39   Existing mature trees

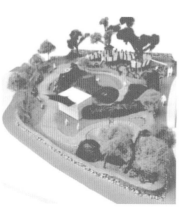

The Royal Cornwall Hospital Trust's Play for Life garden has a "play and healing strategy," balancing various environmental challenges to nurture children's developmental skills.

Orchard Garden Space

This is the therapeutic horticulture and water play space, designed for children to engage to whatever degree they are able with creative & interactive gardening and harvesting activity.
Raised planting beds, accessible from both sides at different levels to suit different abilities provide space for growing and tending flowers and vegetables.
The water ('village') pump and pool basin, surrounded by a sand play space, creates options for plant watering play or free play with water or wet & dry sand.
Planting beds bordering the path contain a rich multisensory range of herbs and fruit bushes, whilst the bank supporting the raised planters is planted with Cornish apple, pear, plum & cherry trees on dwarf rootstocks to enable the full seasonal beauty of the orchard to enhance the users experience.
Sculpture seats set in quiet areas off the path provide scope for intimate seating and observation. The proximity of the garden shelter means that tools for gardening and garden play are easily accessible.
The boundary will be fitted with a protective patterned metal screen showing images of woodland plants & creatures.

1 Ornamental metal gate & boundary screens
2 Woven willow entrance tunnel
3 Willow tunnel
4 Path circuit / trike trail (exposed aggregate concrete)
5 Self binding gravel surface
6 Wooden musical play & carved animals
7 Carved log benches and stools
8 Play hut (recycled existing) store & canopies
9 Apple core space & maze pattern (wet pour surface)
10 Grass rolling bank (mesh reinforced)
11 Play boulder stepping stones & log steps
12 Living willow & hazel poles low hoopped fence
13 Mosaic panel
14 Existing evergreen hedge with chain link fence retained
15 Timber pale fencing
16 Richly multi-sensory planting on banks

Existing path to Tower Block
retained

MH
CL:100.11

Ticket Machine

RCHT Play for Life

Masterplan with Play & Healing Strategy

Introduction

This summary will describe the therapeutic effectiveness of the play design by looking in turn at each of the detailed areas. All areas and play elements are designed to be used by children of all abilities & mobility to different degrees, depending upon their capacity and choice to interact.

The design is intended to offer the clinician / health care worker a range of different sensory, intellectual, social & physical/ mobility options from which to help plan the play experience with the child.

The design is intended to offer a place of respite and sensory richness to both children, teenagers & adults. It is a place with something to offer to everyone in the wider hospital community.

Around the entire site a connecting footpath / trike / scooter / wheelchair trail provides a circuit of movement through a diverse landscape that will entertain, inspire, & absorb the users, taking them out of the hospital environment and into the world of their own imagination.

Singing Ringing Tree Space

This area is designed to offer both free play and quiet retreat. More extensive grass surfacing for free play is surrounded by a range of secluded covered & open areas for relaxation and retreat, using hammock or swing seats, sheltered under willow domes. These elements represent both important swinging motor stimulation as well as psychologically calming environments.

The earth banks surrounding the central lawn will be planted with a rich, multisensory range of natives shrub and herbaceous species (including indigenous fruit trees) to create a wildlife have and viewing opportunity.

The key feature of the whole garden is sited here. The ideas tree' created by the children as part of the consultation program, will be translated into a strikingly beautiful interactive sculpture. It will invite arts workshops to create new ceramic or metal leaves for its branches, which may contain poetry or prose. The tree itself may provide the framework for wind powered sound sculptures.

52 Singing Ringing Tree commemorative sculpture
53 Mesh reinforced turf 'Village green'
54 Sculpture benches
55 Low key self binding gravel circular path
56 Large willow dome furnished with hammock/ swing seat
57 Small willow dome furnished with timber sculpture seats
58 Sloping earth bank, planted with multisensory planting
59 Cornish fruit trees (open shade canopy)

north

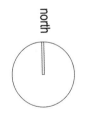

0   1m   5   10   15
bar scale

40 Stone faced hedgebank supporting metal / timber fence & planted trellis
41 Sloping earth bank, planted with multisensory herb and flower planting
42 Cornish fruit trees (open shade canopy)
43 Timber sculpture bench & log seating
44 Wet /dry sand play space (formed concrete haunching)
45 Shallow water basin & pump (formed concrete haunching)
47 Raised bed planters
48 Retained footpath (1800mm) line, kerb & traffic barriers
49 Play hut/ gardener's bothy' store & canopies (exisitng recycled)
50 Activity (wet pour surface) area
51 Self binding gravel area

project:	Play for Life Royal Cornwall Hospital Treliske		
client:	Royal Cornwall Hospital Trust		
drawing:	Masterplan with Play & Healing Strategy		
drg.no.:	PFL-02~14/08/09	r. no.:	
drawn:	-MEW	checked:	-MEW
date:	14/08/09	scale:	1/100 @A1.
notes:	not to used for scaling or scheduling		

westley design
Principal: Michael E. Westley C.M.L.I.
Unit 11 Jubilee Wharf, Commercial Road
Penryn, Cornwall TR10 8FG
tel: +44 (0)1326 259 817, mob: +44 (0)7818 218 879
mike@westleydesign.co.uk
www.westleydesign.co.uk

Warning do not measure or scale! Follow figured dimensions only. If any problems are found or there are any questions about the design please call the number below. This drawing and all design information therein are the property of the Landscape Architect. This drawing may not be reproduced in whole or part without prior written permission from the Landscape Architect.

play, children are also allowed to be quiet, introspective, and to engage in self-discovery. Gardens can be the place to learn conflict resolution skills, find self-confidence, and practice physical skills such as agility and balance. The idea of taking risks may be daunting for children who feel vulnerable and unsafe. The physical play garden environment allows children, at their own pace, to test their physical and psychological parameters, take risks, and gain a new sense of self.

Traditional models of children's playgrounds usually place built elements at the center, leaving nature at the edges of the site. When designing gardens for children who are marginalized, every opportunity to weave the outdoor environment into play must be taken: the response of children to nature's improvisational aspects helps them to build resilience and coping skills, to be creative, and to experience mastery. Nature accommodates without distinction, and children who have felt stigmatized can find acceptance and wonder in the garden. Climbing trees, playing hide and seek in a meadow, or wading and splashing in water are ways to easily engage in spontaneous play with other children. These elements can be incorporated in ways that are available and appealing to all children, regardless of ability. Building connections to others can relieve

Creating art in the garden is a powerful way for children to express their feelings.

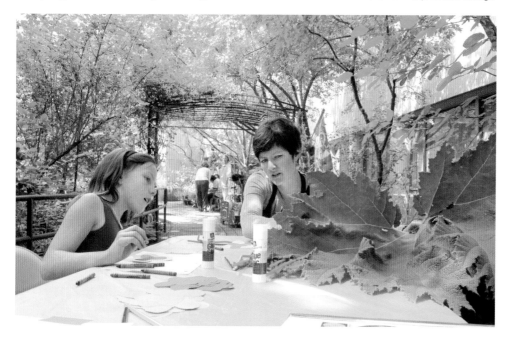

Wire mesh or bamboo poles shaped or lashed together to form teepees or tents can be planted with climbing peas and beans and function as living nooks. Such enclosed retreats offer children a protective sense of peace and serenity.

the loneliness and anxiety associated with trauma and loss. A garden thoughtfully designed to meet these children's needs will be a safe refuge and escape. For many, the garden will give them rare access to nature.

Universal design elements support all children equitably with opportunity for safe, self-directed play and exploration. These types of gardens support success and failure. Graded challenges, such as a series of increasingly difficult climbing elements that begins with a flat path to ambulate on and proceeds to equitable climbing (either on foot or in a wheelchair) can be included. Children can make the decision to use these elements as they choose. These gardens must balance active spaces for children to move around and to express their anger and anxiety in ways that are socially acceptable. Racing up and rolling or stomping down a hill and landing in a bed of sand is a positive way to express negative emotions. Weatherproof easels or tables can be provided with supplies so children can draw and express their feelings through art. There need to be quiet spaces for children, places where they can refocus: small at-grade tree houses, a bean teepee, or a soft bed of grass to lie upon and look up at the lazy clouds.

Gardens for Prison Inmates

The use of gardens in correctional facilities, as places to reform and renew as well as to teach vocational skills, dates back to the late 19th century. Before then, prisoners and those in mental hospitals were treated with routine neglect and isolation. Proponents of moral treatment had a different approach, treating prisoners and those who are mentally ill humanely, with compassion and respect. Moral treatment involved prisoners in tasks associated with daily living, like gardening and farming, as a means of restoring them to a more healthy and meaningful way of life. The integration of mind and body was seen as a path to wellness.

In 1865, Victorian-style gardens were created for and built by prisoners on Alcatraz Island in San Francisco Bay to make the environment more livable. Moral treatment and engagement in purposeful activities like garden installation and gardening enabled prisoners to experience their incarceration at Alcatraz with a degree of dignity, health, and well-being. Now closed as a correctional facility, Alcatraz was an early implementation of a prison reform agenda rising from a strong moral response to increasingly draconian conditions.

Today in many correctional facilities, gardens continue to provide inmates a therapeutic alternative to the lack of perspective and hope that can define incarceration. Instead of passing the time doing little or nothing of personal meaning, inmates at some correctional facilities are provided an opportunity to reconnect with themselves and gain new hope through the rewarding and therapeutic work of tending a garden. One example is the GreenHouse program at Rikers Island Correctional Facility, which is run by the Horticultural Society of New York in collaboration with the NYC Department of Correction and the NYC Department of Education. The Horticultural Society

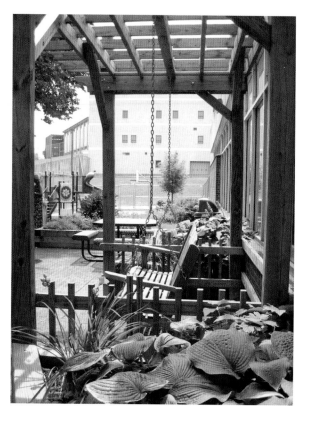

This garden within an enclosed prison courtyard is a safe place for children to play and re-establish bonds with their mothers. The plantings contribute to making the brick patio a peaceful place, where each participant can relax and focus on the short time together.

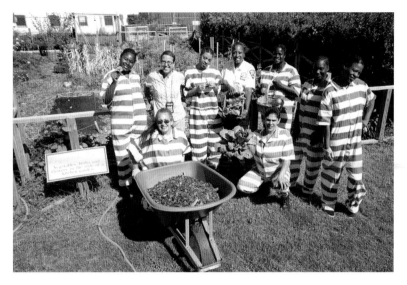

Showing pride and produce at the Green-House program's vegetable patch.

facilitates a program that combines education with horticultural therapy and vocational training, thus offering a positive and productive outlet for inmates. Currently in three different garden spaces, built by inmates and their instructors, one can find landscaped and productive gardens with a greenhouse, classroom buildings, raised bed areas for edibles, and water features. Upon their release from Rikers, graduates of the program can join the GreenTeam, a vocational internship program also sponsored by the Horticultural Society.

The Mother/Child Garden at New York's Bedford Hills Correctional Facility was created in 2005. This maximum security women's facility provides a supportive environment for inmates and their children, who are separated from each other for extensive periods while the mothers serve their sentences. For two weeks every summer, children are transported to the facility for the day. The garden is situated adjacent to the visitor's room with windows that look out into it. At the perimeter of the brick patio are several mature linden trees and three arbors with bench swings, each flanked by raised planters or large pots containing a selection of woodland shrubs and perennials. A large raised bed with wildflowers marks a separation between this space and a large lawn area; across the lawn are a paved basketball court, large play structure, perennial beds, shade trees, and picnic tables.

In the garden, mothers and children meet, play, remember, and reconnect. They cuddle, read, and talk while gently rocking together on the bench swings. Children clamber on play equipment while attended by their mothers, an active connection that is absent for both throughout the rest of the year. The natural setting relieves the stresses of incarceration and separation, and cultivates opportunities for spontaneous and joyful moments for the family. The correctional officers were reluctant at first to embrace the garden, but over time many now value its presence as a calming influence and positive benefit to the Mother/Child program. The garden at Bedford Hills is part of an innovative program that recognizes family and motherhood as a transformative process for female inmates.

Beyond reducing boredom and providing vocational training and opportunities for familial reconnection, gardens for inmates also provide a means of personal survival and connection for political prisoners. Nelson Mandela endured 25 years of incarceration on Robben Island, where the garden provided a thread to life that kept his hopes alive and contributed to his survival; as he wrote in his autobiography, *Long Walk to Freedom*, "A garden is one of the few things in prison that one could control. . . . The sense of being a custodian of this patch of earth offered a small taste of freedom."

DESIGN CONSIDERATIONS

Unlike other user groups, facilitating a participatory design process for a therapeutic garden at a correctional facility poses unique challenges. Inmates are unlikely to be allowed to participate. Instead, a social worker, counselor, warden, or advocate might be willing to share experience and insight with the design team. Other possible resources for the participatory design process are ex-convicts, the formerly homeless, social service providers, or halfway house directors.

One of several basic design guidelines is to use abundant plants, and a great variety of them, to break up the monotony of a prison yard. It is best to avoid red, orange, and bright yellow flowers, since those colors can be associated with anger and hostility. Blues seem to have a calming effect and have been shown to lower blood pressure and reduce fidgety and aggressive behavior (Gruson 1982). Shade is also essential, as hot and overheated inmates may be more inclined to outbursts of anger and to acts of violence. Because privacy is not an option in a correctional facility garden, designing quiet spaces requires creativity and ingenuity. Using different kinds of seating, like boulders and backless benches, enables inmates to choose how they want to sit, which direction to face, and whether to sit upright or be reclined. Offering a degree of choice fosters a sense of self, provides stress relief, and opens the space for self-reflection and assessment.

Gardens for Veterans

In the past many veterans hospitals and long-term recuperation facilities were located in idyllic natural settings. As VA facilities have become massively dense and more urbanized, many have lost their connection to nature and its potential to soften the process of re-entry, provide a desirable place for rehabilitation, and offer relief from the anxieties and stress caused by combat and military service. Today interest is growing in reintegrating nature in the treatment of veterans with physical and psychological wounds.

As veterans of the wars in Iraq and Afghanistan return to the United States with severe polytrauma, treatment facilities are and will be providing long-term physical rehabilitation and psychological services for an increasing number of men and women with devastating injuries such as traumatic brain injury or limb loss, often layered with PTSD. Stress can prolong wound healing, reduce the body's ability to make antibodies, and impair ability to fight infection, and these effects are compounded for those with PTSD by anger, depression, loss of identity, and a sense of hopelessness. Many veterans turn to drugs, alcohol, or other addictive behaviors to seek relief; an alternative form of relief and release is to provide them with access to therapeutic gardens, as they undergo treatment.

At the Walter Reed National Military Medical Center in Bethesda, Maryland, an interdisciplinary team of landscape architects and an occupational therapist prepared design guidelines to redesign the outdoor environments proximal to the therapy clinic and barracks, recommending equitable access to nature for veterans and their families. The overarching idea is to create spaces that are inclusive, meaningful, and purposeful, and which offer, in their variety, ample opportunity for choice. The team determined that a therapeutic garden for veterans would itself be a useful therapeutic intervention as well as a complementary setting for traditional and alternative rehabilitation treatments. Another example of a therapeutic garden design project for veterans, the Warrior and Family Support Center in San Antonio, Texas, provides wounded veterans access to nature with a series of gardens designed by Quatrefoil, Inc. The first phase included multiple courtyards, play areas for children and adults, shade pavilions, and water features. A second phase added trails with varying surfaces and fitness training elements; physical and occupational therapists requested

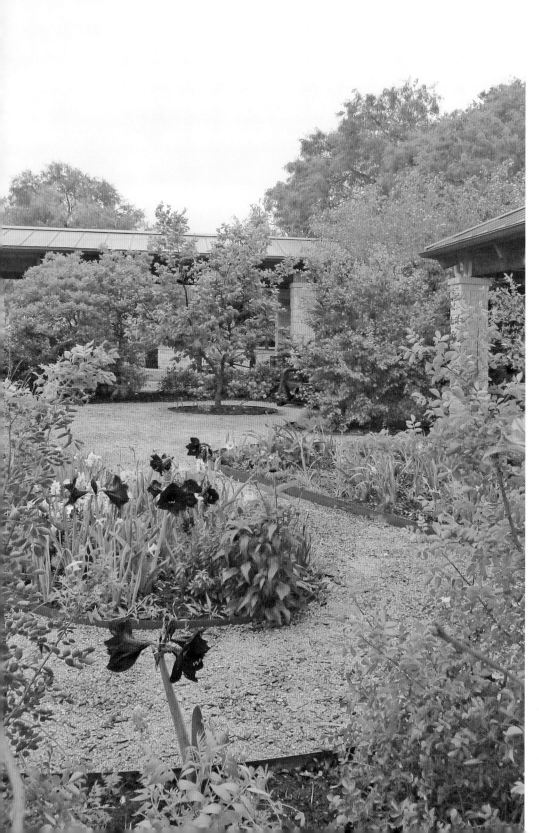

Varied paving
materials in a
terrain park serve as a
realistic rehabilitation
element for veterans
recovering from phys-
ical and emotional
trauma. Richly planted
borders provide
positive distraction
along the way.

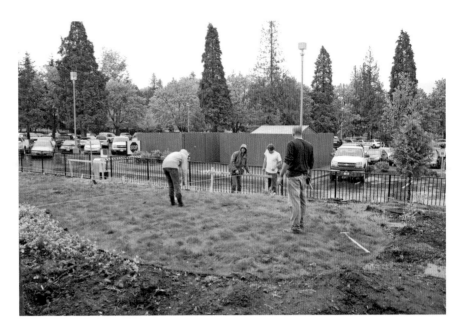

TOP The original landscape at Seattle's Fisher House was a "suburban" archetype—foundation and border shrub plantings and lawn—surrounded by parking lot. Transforming it into a therapeutic garden began with intense site planning.

BOTTOM A subtly demarcated space furnished with a swing and views into the garden offers veterans and their family members a place to think and reflect in highly charged situations. The swing's gentle rocking motion has a soothing stress-reduction effect.

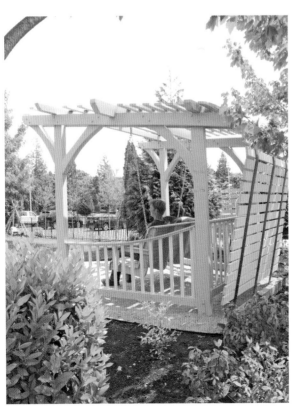

these as realistic settings in which to address community reintegration skills.

In another two-phase project, students from University of Washington's landscape architecture design/build studio partnered with VA Puget Sound Health to create therapeutic gardens for veterans at the Fisher House in Seattle. The students redesigned the entire site in two phases, starting with lawn removal. From the house's communal kitchen, a series of French doors now opens onto a patio and outdoor living room. Wide and level sensory walking paths loop around the house, leading to pavilions for yoga and meditation, arbors, bench swings, a children's playscape, universally accessible vegetable gardens, and a small waterfall. The therapeutic gardens extend a sense of home, of refuge, to veterans undergoing treatment, as well as to their families, who live at Fisher House during this stressful time. Anecdotal findings since the final phase was completed have been unequivocally positive. "This really is a healing garden," one guest reflected. "I sat on a bench, and I started to cry. I didn't know I needed to cry, but it felt so good when I was done. What a beautiful place."

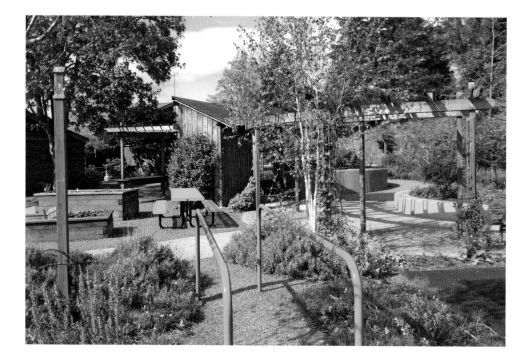

DESIGN CONSIDERATIONS

Because gardens for veterans serve both veterans and their families, they should offer multigenerational appeal. Playful sensory elements—freestanding musical chimes, talking tubes, tabletop and at-grade game boards—offer positive distraction for children. For families waiting for a veteran's appointment to end, an inviting garden to retreat to can make the seemingly eternal waits feel shorter and more pleasant. Spaces for privacy and places for fun and socializing, including a barbeque area, need to be thoughtfully located and sequenced within the site. Elements that support physical rehabilitation such as steps, parallel bars, and ramps will accentuate the usefulness of these gardens, whether they are located where such services are offered or in a park within proximity of a hospital or rehabilitation clinic. Night lighting will extend the garden's benefits, allowing users to sit outside and quietly visit or read.

The concept of using gardens as both immersive and programmatic therapeutic tools to assist veterans and their families during recovery from illness and reentry into the community is relatively new for patients and therapists. As the military explores effective means of healing and reconnection, the role of environmental design is receiving attention from administrators and physicians, lending support to the idea that more gardens will be planned and integrated into military facilities.

Traditional indoor physical rehabilitation modalities like parallel bars can be integrated into a therapeutic garden for veterans.

Gardens for Immigrants

Culturally relevant gardens play an important role in reconnecting people with their roots. The casita represents an oasis within an intensely urban, paved environment, where even a stand of Japanese knotweed is welcomed for its breezy tropical air.

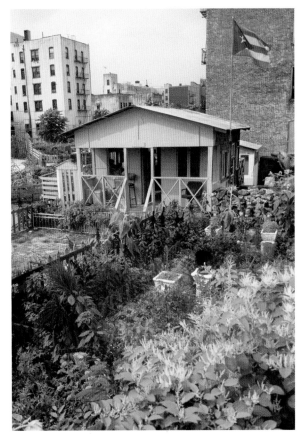

Whether legal or undocumented, immigrants often endure poverty, trauma, forced displacement, and unemployment. The impacts of immigration resonate in communities worldwide. People who are displaced can experience a profound sense of loss, confusion, and depression as they strive to forge lives in new places that are difficult to decipher and navigate, and that may feel very unwelcoming. Plants are instrumental components of place; certain plants vividly recall former homes, and by tending them in a new place, a new garden, immigrants can simultaneously put down roots in their new home and pass their memories on to their children.

In New York City, in the 1970s, immigrants arriving from Puerto Rico were presented with a unique opportunity: their housing projects lacked close access to parks but nearby vacant lots were abundant. With incredible ingenuity and thrift and much experience of building and planting, these immigrants transformed overlooked sites into their "home" landscapes. They hauled in soil, salvaged wood and tin from abandoned buildings, had seeds sent from Puerto Rico, and created casitas ("little houses"), intensely expressive community gardens. Examples of casita gardens have been documented in Philadelphia, Chicago, Boston, and many other large industrial cities.

These gardens reconnected Puerto Rican immigrants to memories of the vibrant green island of their youth and helped restore their well-being, optimism, and confidence. The recreated landscape was a distraction from marginalization, menial jobs, and the emotional struggles that attended them as they coped with change in a troubled urban environment. For these immigrants, the casita was a refuge, where the familiarity of spaces, built forms, rituals, and artistic expression created a safe place to reestablish their

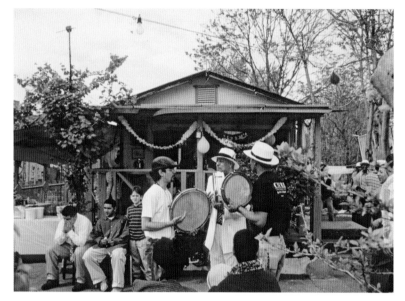

Much of life in Puerto Rico is focused on music, and this connection to place and people is fostered in the casita.

identity and look to the future. In a similar manner, African Americans who moved from the rural south to northern cities in the Great Migration created gardens reminiscent of their former home gardens. When civil rights were being contested, and the "Black power" and "Latino pride" movements were flourishing, these culturally rich gardens functioned as centers of community solidarity.

In 2013, a keyhole garden was installed at the Guatemalan-Maya Center, which provides social services to the many Guatemalan Mayan refugees who live and work in Lake Worth, Florida. First developed in drought-ridden areas of Africa and used extensively in Guatemala, keyhole gardens combine accessibility with environmental sustainability and return on investment. They are circular, usually constructed of stone or other easily found objects, and typically about six feet in diameter, but they can be built to a height of choice to accommodate the widest range of users. There is a wedge notched out of the circle and a hole in the center of the circle, where a compost basket that is about a foot higher than the walls of the garden is placed. An aerial view reveals the open wedge and central composting basket in the shape of a keyhole, hence its name. Standing in the wedge or at the outer wall allows the gardener access to all points, so every bit of the garden is available for planting. Of note though:

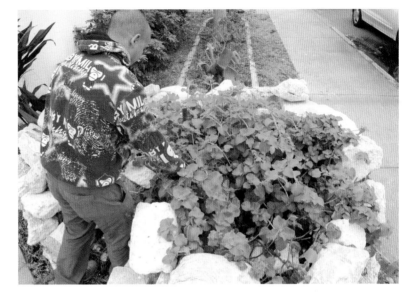

For the Guatemalan Mayan community in south Florida, the keyhole garden is an iconic memory of home. This one is planted with Mexican mint (*Plectranthus amboinicus*).

the form is not ergonomically well designed for seated gardeners, who must sit sideways, which is stressful to the body.

The ability of vernacular gardens, including casitas, traditional African American home gardens, and keyhole gardens, to provide therapeutic benefits to their makers/users has been documented anecdotally and through ethnographic research; and the need for further design and creation of such gardens, which have a unique capacity to strengthen a distinct minority's cultural identity, is great. The lessons learned from vernacular gardens can help future designers create culturally relevant gardens for schoolyards, community centers, and social service and health facilities that serve immigrant and refugee communities.

DESIGN CONSIDERATIONS

Gardens for immigrants are usually created through grassroots efforts. In order to ensure that these gardens foster positive memories for the community they are meant to serve, a high degree of sensitivity is required on the part of the design team. It is imperative to listen to the needs of the community and to research their culture, to understand the complexity and stresses caused by their transition and how nature can alleviate the unhealthful effects of this process. If language is a barrier, use interpreters (often a younger family member) and consider facilitating language-free (or language-limited) workshop processes, such as card-sorts or inviting users to use stickers to rank images they like or dislike. Consider referencing positive archetypes of the homeland, using symbols that foster positive memories. This must be done carefully, as many immigrants may be fleeing from traumatic situations, and their memories are filled with fear and shame. The Internet is a readily available resource, and many cities have cultural heritage centers that can provide information about the cultural and/or ethnic group you are designing for.

Universal design features will extend a welcome to the entire community: the elderly, the younger generation, those with and those without physical, intellectual, and emotional challenges. It is important that those who live near the garden are included, so that bridges of friendship and respect are formed and any negative feelings assuaged before they escalate. The garden must be easily comprehensible, and an instructor or mentor may be needed to guide new participants. The feeling of safety is critical, especially when language barriers prevent users from feeling connected to their community and to the garden; any signage should include simple and universal icons in addition to words.

Because the sense of displacement and lack of control is common among immigrants, the garden must offer its users a sense of ownership. In a production garden, users should have a raised bed, pot, or row or two in the garden to call their own. If the intent is more passive, inviting users to design their own tile for a mosaic wall or to take turns maintaining the garden increases self-empowerment and the sense of ownership and belonging. The design should include spaces and activities where users connect with each other and to the land. If possible, create conditions where people can grow familiar plants and create places where traditional celebrations can take place.

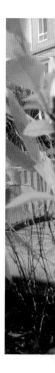

Gardens for the Homeless

The homeless represent another marginalized group who may reap the benefits of access to therapeutic gardens. Catastrophic health problems, compounded with unemployment, are a common route to loss of place and home, although causes and conditions of homelessness are varied, complex, and multilayered. Many homeless people have been traumatized by sexual abuse or other violence; many struggle with substance abuse or are mentally ill. A therapeutic garden, especially in an urban area, can be a safe and calm place to reengage, reconnect, and relearn skills that support the transition to stability and self-sufficiency. Designers can find opportunities to work with the homeless through transitional and permanent housing programs. These housing models can readily integrate therapeutic gardens, whether with at-grade open spaces or on rooftops. Most housing for the homeless is being developed by nonprofit social service agencies and federal- and state-funded groups.

At the Village Spirit Center for Community Change and Healing in Seattle, predominantly black families are provided permanent housing, vocational training, education, and counseling. The funder, Catholic Community Services of Western Washington, acknowledges and embraces the spirituality, cultural relevance, and celebration of the black community, and the block-long therapeutic garden, situated on a central intergenerational rooftop courtyard, is an important component of the transitional process from uncertainty and homelessness to stability. The design concept strings four garden rooms linearly along the axis of the courtyard and extends the family and community life inside the apartments out into the landscape, successfully integrating children's playscape, social spaces, exercise zones, and reflection garden. Each family also has their own raised planter just outside their front door. The first of the four rooms is devoted

Designing to encourage a meaningful connection to place can be enhanced through understanding the culture of the user group. The curved seating area is a sanctuary, reminiscent of the circular clearings in the woods where slaves once prayed.

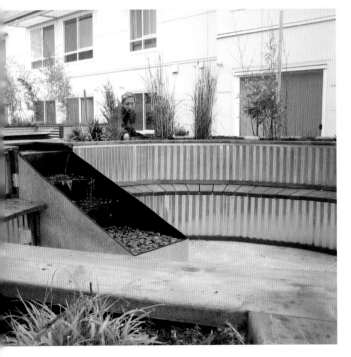

to urban farm cultivation beds with a food preparation and cooking area. The second, a community "living room," features an arbor with a movie screen and terraced seating for community meetings and celebrations; it is also a place for enjoying a barbeque and roasting vegetables harvested from the residents' raised planters. The third, a sanctuary element, is an inward-focused refuge where parents and their children can sit on the curved seats and enjoy the sounds of a burbling water feature, surrounded by ornamental grasses waving in the breeze.

The fourth room is a playscape designed for intergenerational recreation and learning. Simple climbable mounds interspersed on level ADA matting increase its flexibility. The open circulation is intentional and

An element like a map of the neighborhood serves multiple purposes. It orients users and provides connection to their new home and nearby community. It is also a fun element for children to run, skip, hop, or ride bicycles or trikes along.

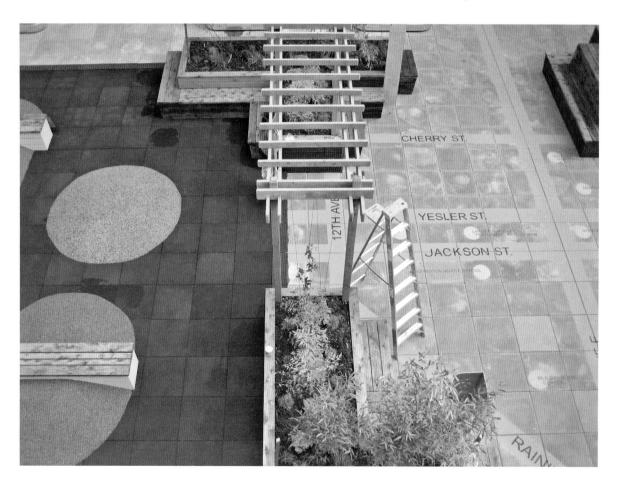

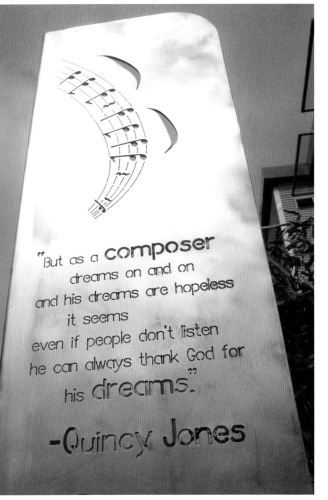

Totems honoring local people whose work and legacy have helped to shape a community have an important place in a garden designed to support reflection and remembrance.

encourages social interaction; children wheel and play throughout the safe, enclosed courtyard while their parents watch them and interact with other families.

During the participatory design process, residents asked that African Americans who had contributed to the cultural life of Seattle's black community be honored somehow. Accordingly, eight iconic totems were placed throughout the garden, each honoring the legacy of an important African American in the Pacific Northwest. The totems inspire pride in the residents, many of whom have low self-esteem and self-worth due to issues of homelessness, unemployment, and abuse.

The Homeless Garden Project in Santa Cruz, California, is another example of a garden that builds bridges and weaves the homeless population into the local community. It is freestanding, created to address the needs of a transient population, and is not associated with transitional or permanent housing. The garden is based on a model that views gardening as a meaningful and productive endeavor, one that supports the learning, sharing, and practice of vocational and life skills. It was conceived as a business (those who are homeless sell their harvest to local restaurants and farmers' markets) and has transitioned into a thriving CSA (community supported agriculture) model. Local community members buy produce, herbs, and flowers from the project's gardeners, and the garden serves to reconnect the gardeners to their former communities. The Homeless Garden Project is a replicable model; visit homelessgardenproject.org to learn more.

Based in West Palm Beach, Florida, The Lord's Place is a nonprofit, nonsectarian organization whose mission is to break the cycle of homelessness through innovative services for men, women, and children. One of the programs at The Lord's Place is the Urban Garden, a venue for learning real-life vocational skills while actively engaging with nature; its accessible production garden exemplifies the farm-to-fork model.

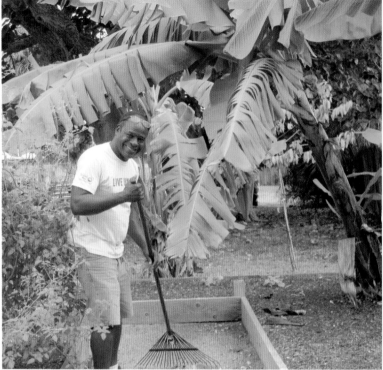

Tending production gardens at homeless organizations fosters a sense of self-worth and self-sufficiency in clients.

Vegetables and herbs grown in the garden are used by apprentices in the culinary arts training program; they in turn prepare food served at an onsite café, which feeds the needy on a daily basis and provides catering services to local businesses. Produce is also sold to local restaurants and at green markets. Whether they are designed as freestanding or as part of a transitional housing facility, therapeutic gardens for those experiencing homelessness are very empowering: as one new gardener put it, "What I have learned about being and working in the garden is that I can forget about what happened in the past and concentrate on what is happening now."

DESIGN CONSIDERATIONS

Designing gardens for the homeless requires sensitivity, honesty, openness, and empathy. Most people have little direct experience with this marginalized population, and many designers may unwittingly bring personal and societal stereotypes to the project. As always, a participatory design process is the best way to gain insight into the needs, hopes, and preferences of these underserved people. In cases where access is restricted and cultural/communication barriers must be overcome, an "expert" may have to suffice in lieu of the actual users.

Establish active spaces by including a production or working garden. Because users will range widely in age and ability, a variety of at-grade and fully accessible raised beds will allow most if not all to participate in tending and maintaining the garden. Paths need to be at least three feet wide, enough to accommodate one wheeled mobility device, and ideally are formed from tinted concrete. Mulch is the least desirable option, even if the budget is tight; no matter the type of garden it is installed in, it is hard to wheel over and walk on, particularly for those with impaired mobility. Paths should be cleared of debris and free of cracks, and raised beds and planters free of splinters, sharp edges, or cracks to avoid unforeseen injuries.

Multigenerational activities may need to be an integral part of gardens for the homeless, as all too often entire families are affected. Adults who are working in or socializing at the garden need to know that their children have a safe and novel place to play and explore. Sightlines between the garden and children's play spaces must be clear and unobstructed so adults can adequately supervise their children. For any adult, mentoring younger children improves their sense of self-worth, of being a useful member of the community, and it may rekindle fond memories of raising their own children; when multiple generations work and play together, the young ask questions and stories emerge about family histories. Establishing a set of rules (for example, no running or riding toys in the garden) will keep young and seasoned gardeners safer by avoiding any potential collisions. Seating needs to be located so older adults can sit, tell stories, or read a book to the younger participants. Fencing or other types of containment will keep children inside the garden area and unwanted guests out. All garden tools need to be kept out of young children's reach, as do any chemicals (although it is better not to use any). Amenities such as shade, water, safe storage for tools and bags, and restrooms will enhance the comfort and usability of the garden for this marginalized group.

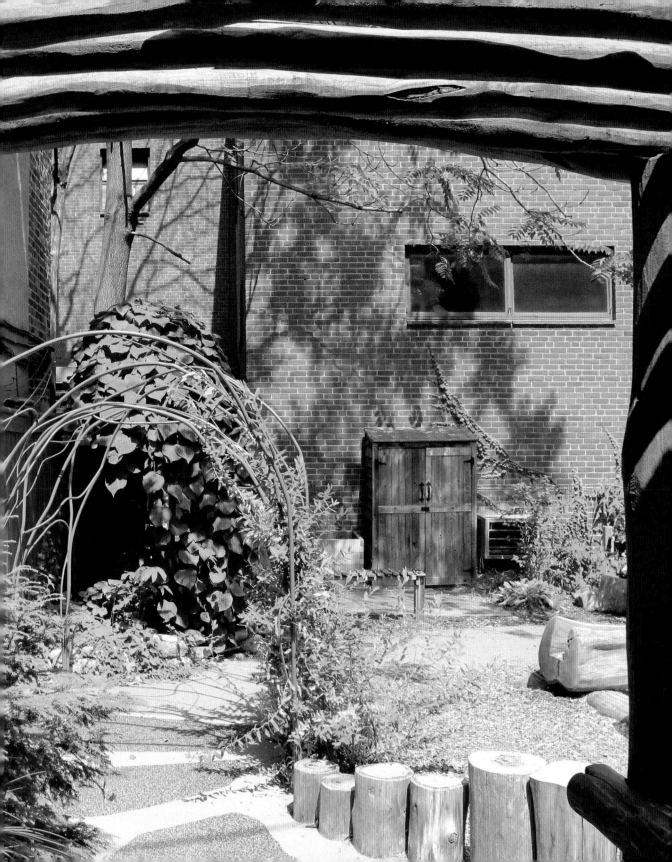

CHAPTER FIVE
LEARNING GARDENS

Therapeutic gardens that support learning in traditional and non-traditional places can be transformative. The skills acquired in them go beyond basic academic knowledge and on into life lessons, like cooperation, resilience, patience, reaching beyond one's comfort level, and connection with others as well as the earth. Learning extends beyond simply tending plants; a learning garden can complement an indoor classroom as an alternative place to hold classes, lectures, discussions, storytelling, and activity groups. Being in nature improves attentional capacity and focus, and learning outdoors nurtures curiosity, exploration, and discovery. Those benefiting from learning gardens include children with cognitive (intellectual) disabilities or who have limited exposure to nature; intergenerational groups bridging differences; disparate groups seeking to reconnect, mediate conflict, or confront traumatic events; and people, often marginalized or underserved, looking to learn new vocational skills.

A learning garden is a place where participants learn about and care for plants. Learning takes place in a nonthreatening environment, and all participants, regardless of physical and cognitive abilities, are accepted and embraced. Most people are genuinely pleased when a seed they planted sprouts, when a plant they propagated grows, flowers, and bears fruit. Providing seating, shade, water (for humans and plants), planting beds at various heights, and accessible, smooth, well-drained, wide paths are essential to all learning gardens. Providing garden tools that meet the diverse needs of all potential users increases the usability of the garden and enables more people to participate.

Shared by a teacher and school garden coordinator: The most valuable thing about teaching in the garden and other outdoor classroom areas is that it is a great equalizer for students. Even if they are struggling academically, they can be successful in the garden. They develop self-confidence while learning healthy eating habits and create a connection to their food source and the environment. If we expect our students to become the future stewards of the earth, they need to develop a love for and connection to it.

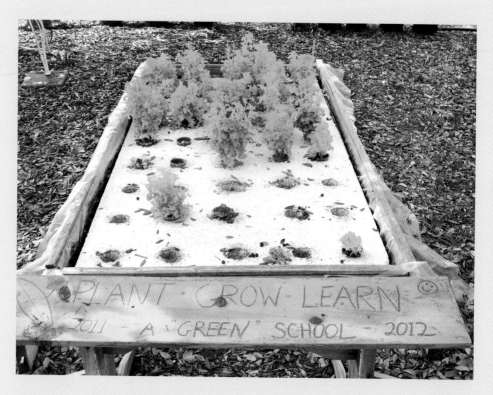

Plant, grow, learn—and smile—in a garden. When plants thrive, their primary stewards do as well.

Outdoor Classrooms

At the VA Puget Sound Fisher House, raised beds at various heights provide choices for gardeners to safely kneel, sit, or stand to garden.

Florida's Palm Beach County School District is the 11th largest in the United States. From 2009 to 2013, the district, in partnership with a grant from the Robert Wood Johnson Foundation (and matching funding), made significant environmental changes in some of their lowest-income schools. Poverty and food insecurity impact every school in the Lake Worth, Palm Springs, and Greenacres area of the county (where, according to the county healthcare district's annual BMI study, more than 45 percent of the students at one school were obese in 2010). All schools in this sector were offered a chance to create a Healthy Kids, Healthy Communities garden on their site. Many of the students speak English as a second language, and they or their parents emigrated from Latin America or the

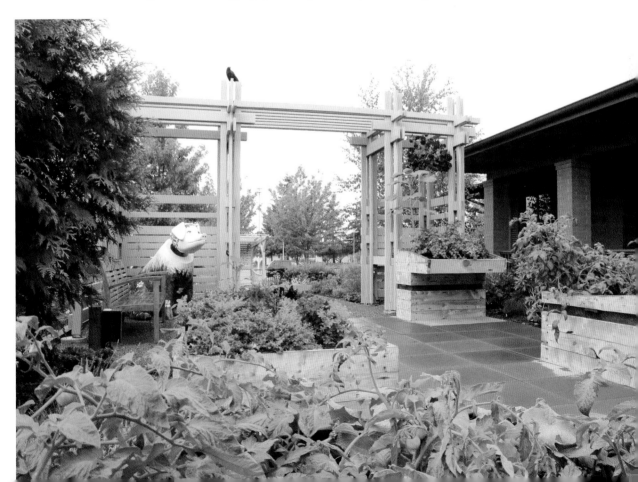

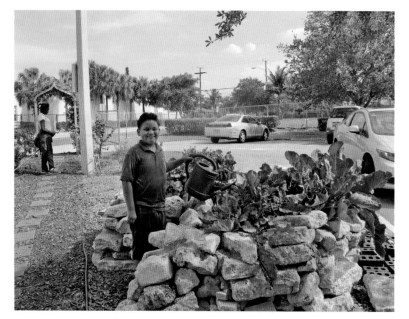

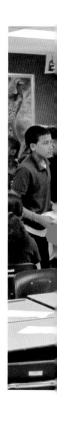

At South Grade Elementary in Lake Worth, a vernacular keyhole garden is a nod to the school's large population of Guatemalan Mayan students. Designed at a height comfortable for children, it is a popular spot in the garden.

Caribbean. Most of the 30 school and community neighborhood gardens funded through the grant celebrate the children's cultural roots by planting vegetables and herbs associated with their countries of origin.

The positive outcomes are evident to whoever visits, children and adults alike. A change comes over the students when they are outside among the plants they have been learning about and tending. Children are thrilled to be given the responsibility of watering or planting a seed, and check back regularly to measure the growth of the plants and see the small animals that visit their garden every day. For many, the greatest reward comes when they harvest the fruits of their labor. Most cannot wait, and eat what they are picking before they leave the garden. Children who never tried a pepper argue over who found the biggest and who can eat it the fastest. Over in Greenacres, teacher Ted Gliptis draws on his former experience in the food industry to take students at Forest Hill Elementary from growing fruit and vegetables in the courtyard garden to cooking and eating what is harvested. What is not relished in the garden or classroom is shared with others in the school, or packed up and sent home with the enthusiastic young growers.

Each garden is a significant asset for the teachers who volunteer as

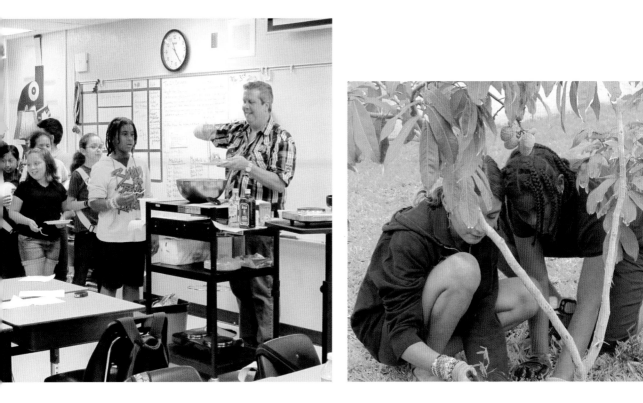

garden coordinators. All the gardens have become an extension of the school curriculum and provide teachers a creative alternative to educate their students in ways that bring them out of the traditional classroom setting to explore the merits of hands-on learning. At any time during the day or after school, children and teachers are outside cultivating, weeding, and harvesting vegetables, doing scientific investigations, writing stories, sketching, identifying plants, insects, and butterflies, and learning to work together in small and large groups. What is learned in these gardens cultivates future environmental stewardship and important life lessons such as understanding the life cycles and principles of sustainability. According to grant coordinator Erica Whitfield, the new attitude in Palm Beach County is that every school should have a garden.

Access to nature positively influences cognitive skills. For some children, access may be limited because of movement challenges, such as those associated with juvenile rheumatoid arthritis or developmental disabilities like cerebral palsy or, compounded with intellectual disability, Down syndrome. Others may fear being outside because of lack of experience. Parental fears about nature play or children's preference for indoor play can also explain why some children lack immersive nature experiences. Children who live in marginalized neighborhoods are least likely to have access to safe, outdoor environments, diminishing their opportunities to benefit and learn from the moderating and positive effects of nature. Whether it is intrinsic or extrinsic factors that prevent access to nature, learning gardens can be designed to support all children, regardless of their ability or experience.

Gardens are ideal environments to refine specific learning skills for children or adults with developmental disabilities in purposeful and engaging ways. For instance, tasking someone to fill each of eight baskets with 10 ripe tomatoes starts with identifying ripe tomatoes and counting. Comparing and contrasting the physical properties of different tomato cultivars entails investigative scientific and observational skills as well as language skills. Visual, perceptual, and spatial skills are tapped: how can 10 tomatoes fit into the basket without falling out? There are motor-movement benefits, as the gardener bends up and down, harvesting the fruit. Picking tomatoes involves touch, smell, taste, sight, and even pro-prioception and kinesthesia (more on these in chapter 6), to calculate the proper amount of pressure needed to pick only the tomato and not disturb the plant. With renewed interest in social enterprise, learning gardens offer "fertile ground" for learning and applying business skills by growing, harvesting, packaging, and managing the operation of selling products.

Outdoor classrooms are effective ways to introduce children to nature through inquiry and directed play exploration. A classroom is a controlled environment, and children with intellectual challenges or with little experience with (or fear of) nature may find this environment a secure setting in which to explore and connect with nature and themselves. Outdoor classrooms are often aligned with schools, camps, communities, or environmental centers. Universal design principles will thoughtfully accommodate children of varying abilities and experience. Defining the classroom by signaling a transition into the space will denote the area as a place of learning, setting it apart from activities abutting it. Boundaries, including changes in paving and surfaces, hedges, fruit-bearing trees, vertical gardens, raised beds, or attractive fencing, will also prepare children to focus inward on the natural world of the classroom. The living walls thus become integral components of the learning experience as students water and tend them. Flowers, leaves, and fruits can be counted and categorized. Children can photograph or draw pictures of the walls in different seasons, comparing and contrasting similar and dissimilar features.

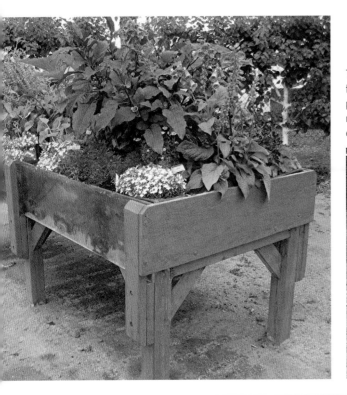

This raised bed allows seated gardeners to directly face and work the bed, an important ergonomic principle, and to observe the growing process from roots through fruit, which heightens the learning experience and inspires curiosity.

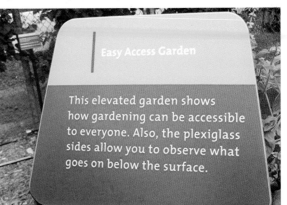

Easy Access Garden

This elevated garden shows how gardening can be accessible to everyone. Also, the plexiglass sides allow you to observe what goes on below the surface.

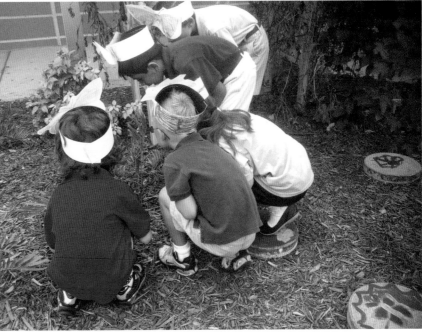

Observing stem and leaf physiology firsthand optimizes and carries over the indoor learning process.

An outdoor classroom must be a flexible space, serving as a science lab in the morning and a creative writing room after lunch. Flexibility necessitates that the space be open, shaded, and uncluttered, and storage be provided for garden tools and supplies, hose bibs, and portable seating. Classroom facilitators and children define how the space is used. Opportunities to learn individually or as a group should be embedded in the design. A flexible gathering space can be furnished with portable chairs and lap desks, a rolling chalk- or whiteboard, and space for wheeled mobility devices. Smaller ancillary spaces with tunnels, tree stumps, tree houses, and patches of soft grass enable children to find their own quiet sanctuaries to do their work.

For those uncertain about physically connecting with nature (e.g., sitting on the grass or a tree stump), sturdy folding stools become the intermediaries between formal seating and immersive contact. In time and with increased exposure, these children may explore a more direct physical and cerebral connection with nature. For children who use mobility devices, ample space to wheel around and be close to other children is necessary.

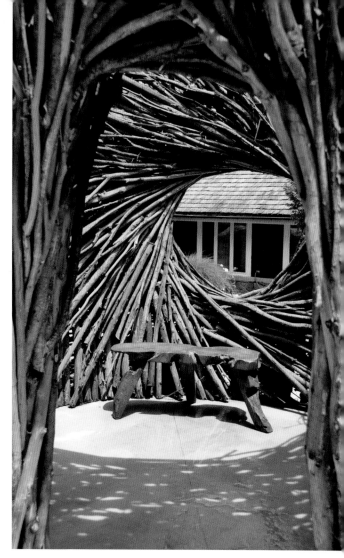

A bentwood structure provides a measure of shelter from the elements and is a quiet place to work.

LEARNING RINGS FOR CHILDREN WITH INTELLECTUAL DISABILITIES

Learning rings or stations are an organized system to support directed and self-guided experiences. The concept is applicable to outdoor classrooms but can also be incorporated into any therapeutic garden design. Whether they are designed as a single-loop space or as concentric rings, learning rings support structured learning experiences while nurturing self-discovery. Both designs support cooperative learning.

The government-funded Marnebek School, on the southeastern edge of Melbourne, Australia, serves five- to 18-year-olds with mild to profound intellectual disability. Children with intellectual disabilities learn differently from their typically developing peers, and some may also have movement challenges. They may need more time to learn a concept. They may require increased assistance from others to learn, often

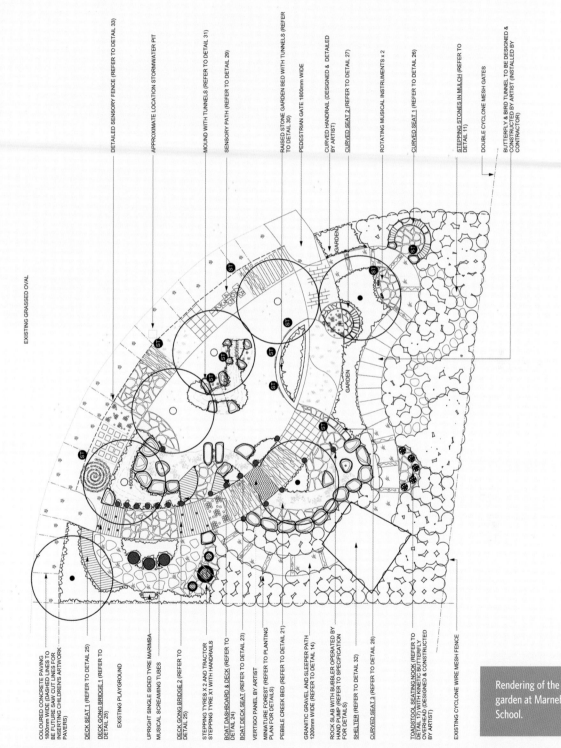

EXISTING GRASSED OVAL

DETAILED SENSORY FENCE (REFER TO DETAIL 33)

APPROXIMATE LOCATION STORMWATER PIT

MOUND WITH TUNNELS (REFER TO DETAIL 31)

SENSORY PATH (REFER TO DETAIL 29)

RAISED STONE GARDEN BED WITH TUNNELS (REFER TO DETAIL 30)

PEDESTRIAN GATE 1800mm WIDE

CURVED HANDRAIL (DESIGNED & DETAILED BY ARTIST)

CURVED SEAT 2 (REFER TO DETAIL 27)

ROTATING MUSICAL INSTRUMENTS x 2

CURVED SEAT 1 (REFER TO DETAIL 26)

STEPPING STONES IN MULCH (REFER TO DETAIL 11)

DOUBLE CYCLONE MESH GATES

BUTTERFLY & BIRD TUNNEL, TO BE DESIGNED & CONSTRUCTED BY ARTIST (INSTALLED BY CONTRACTOR)

COLOURED CONCRETE PAVING 1800mm WIDE (DASHED LINES TO BE FUTURE SAW CUT LINES FOR INSERTING CHILDREN'S ARTWORK PAVERS)

DECK SEAT 1 (REFER TO DETAIL 25)

DECK GONG BRIDGE 1 (REFER TO DETAIL 25)

EXISTING PLAYGROUND

UPRIGHT SINGLE SIDED TYRE MARIMBA

MUSICAL SCREAMING TUBES

DECK GONG BRIDGE 2 (REFER TO DETAIL 25)

STEPPING TYRES X 2 AND TRACTOR STEPPING TYRE X1 WITH HANDRAILS

BOAT DASHBOARD & DECK (REFER TO DETAIL 24)

BOAT DECK SEAT (REFER TO DETAIL 23)

VERTIGO PANEL BY ARTIST

MINIATURE FOREST (REFER TO PLANTING PLAN FOR DETAILS)

PEBBLE CREEK BED (REFER TO DETAIL 21)

GRANITIC GRAVEL AND SLEEPER PATH 1200mm WIDE (REFER TO DETAIL 14)

ROCK SLAB WITH BUBBLER OPERATED BY HAND PUMP (REFER TO SPECIFICATION FOR DETAILS)

SHELTER (REFER TO DETAIL 32)

CURVED SEAT 3 (REFER TO DETAIL 28)

TOADSTOOL SEATING NOOK (REFER TO DETAIL 17) WITH KINETIC BUTTERFLY OVERHEAD (DESIGNED & CONSTRUCTED BY ARTIST)

EXISTING CYCLONE WIRE MESH FENCE

Rendering of the garden at Marnebek School.

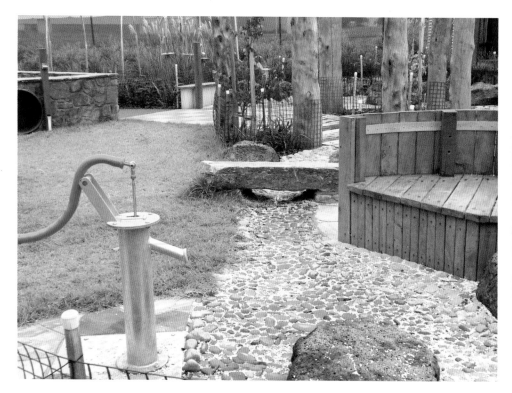

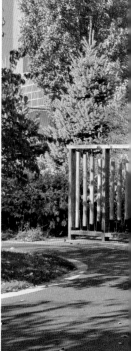

needing intensive repetition, or a combination of sensory modalities, like watching, listening, and doing. Accommodating these varying modes of learning requires flexible workspaces. The goal at Marnebek was to create an outdoor space exceeding the needs of its diverse population, a space where students could find activities, spaces, and qualities in the environment to meet their particular needs.

The new garden complements the school's standard outdoor play equipment, providing much-needed alternatives for the students and offering a wide range of sensory experiences and enrichment opportunities for individual and group play and for therapy. The planting articulates a series of "rooms" as well as functioning as a wind buffer. Textured paths and fencing are contrasted and complemented by the natural colors and textures of the planting palette. Students can view natural light through colored translucent panels and artworks and listen to and make music. Interactive sound and art sculptures and other tactile sensory experiences enrich or desensitize those who are overstimulated. Other features support social interaction and learning, including speaker tubes, the pumping action required to feed the stream, and fully accessible squeaky tires that encourage jumping, balancing, playing, and laughing. Response to the garden, designed in 2006 by Jeavons Landscape Architects (then Mary Jeavons Landscape Architects), has been overwhelmingly positive.

One way science can be brought into an outdoor classroom is to have students measure the volume of water pumped in a specific amount of time. Note the hidey hole in the left corner, where a child can go to be or work alone, or watch such inquiries from afar.

Designing raised beds that children or adults can sit at (or roll under, if using a wheelchair) without twisting their bodies is an important ergonomic principle.

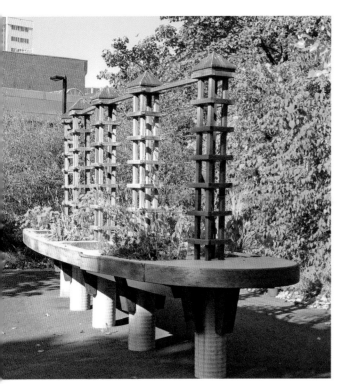

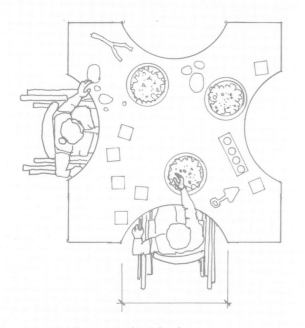

An example of how a group of seated gardeners can work together in a way that is ergonomically correct, thus reducing stress on their bodies.

DESIGN CONSIDERATIONS

A facilitator closely supervises, directs, and teaches student(s) from the core of a concentric rings design. Arranged around the central core, individual beds encourage children to work individually under the facilitator's watchful eye and develop social skills as they interact and learn from one another. A removable-covered trough or cantilevered garden that wheeled mobility users can roll under and others can sit or stand at is well suited as the anchor of the learning garden and encourages diverse interactions. Uncovered, it is a place where children can engage in plant-related learning activities; covered, it becomes a space for traditional learning experiences like mathematical exercises, writing, or drawing plants.

An inherent design challenge: a cover could very well crush the plants. The lid must be constructed to fit over the trough and above the plants. A flat lid would be too high for a child to use in a functional or comfortable manner. Can you imagine having to reach up and over a barrier (like the lid) to write or draw? A simple solution is to create a fold-down lid to fit over the trough. From an ergonomic perspective, this design is advantageous for anyone. Writing at a 30- to 45-degree angle allows children to rest their forearms on the work surface. This setup reduces stress on the shoulder and arm joints, and positions the arm comfortably to write or draw.

At each successive ring, the learning experiences become more challenging but sequenced so the children can, as appropriate, direct their own activities rather than be directed by a facilitator. Moving beyond the central core demonstrates increasing competence. Design elements that encourage more complex learning challenges include rings of raised beds that the children are individually responsible to care for. The beds can be large planters with secure bases, individual trough gardens, or grow bags set on tables or at grade. The living surround or walls of an outdoor classroom are at the perimeter; these vertical elements represent another opportunity to learn about different types of plantings.

LEARNING RINGS FOR CHILDREN WITH LIMITED EXPOSURE TO NATURE

Learning ring design also introduces children to and supports those with limited exposure to nature. For those fearful of natural elements like insects or snakes, getting dirty, or of the physical challenges of climbing or gardening, these rings offer enticing activities conducive to the child's current level of development.

DESIGN CONSIDERATIONS

A learning ring with a single loop design feels less intimidating and self-contained to children with limited exposure to nature, and because loops never end, there is no getting lost. The stations of the learning ring are sequenced from simple to complex. A level and grassy area located in the center of the loop houses the staging and compost hub (the composting zone is separated from the stations so those with mold allergies will not be affected). Compost bins should be small enough that children can experience a direct connection with the process of decomposition; multiple bins enable children to participate in the composting activities simultaneously. The hub also houses soil, buckets, pots, carts, and other garden tools and supplies that support the learning stations while "class" is in session, though adequate storage space for tools and toys should be nearby. Unlike a concentric ring design, a single loop allows children to slowly navigate a logical sequence of graded nature-based activities that offer compatible challenges; in a graded concept, outdoor experiences increase in modest increments, intensity, and complexity. Little by little, children learn to explore beyond their comfort zone in an environment that feels safe, engenders a sense of control, and presents appropriate challenges. The spectrum of activities ranges from highly structured to self-directed and is manageable, interesting, and not so difficult as to be insurmountable and trigger frustration or fear. The challenges, also on a gradient, range from passive, observational activities to hands-on learning endeavors that support structured active participation.

For safety reasons the learning rings must be surrounded by secure fencing and designed for unobstructed visibility looking out from and into the garden. Like outdoor classrooms, they should be located close to schools, community centers, family homeless shelters, and faith-based facilities. Easy access is necessary so that children can be gently coaxed out to the learning garden and the transition is easy, without distraction or confusion. The garden can actually "begin" inside the building and gradually transition out into the garden. A view of the outdoor classroom is a passive introduction, preparing and encouraging children to venture outside. Accessible window boxes or movable plant trolleys filled with inviting plants, magnifying lenses, and water misters, used inside, are other small, introductory steps to the great outdoors. Engaging wayfinding—a "stepping stone" path of vinyl sunflower or daisy decals affixed to the floor—will gently lead children to the doorway and into the learning garden.

Natural elements such as upended logs carved to become chairs subtly connect even reluctant children with nature.

In the first space, passive and observational learning is supported. Seating constructed with natural materials faces into the garden and invites children to watch until they are ready to venture into the garden. Hollowed-out bench logs, tree stumps, and child-sized bentwood rocking chairs are ways to connect children with nature.

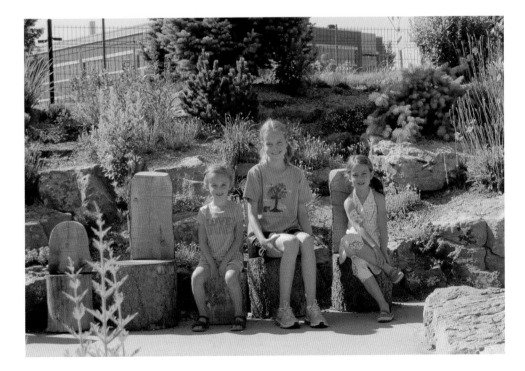

A space with multiple pairs of child-sized binoculars encourages observation; identifying birds snacking from feeders oriented around the ring is a provocative entry exercise. Raised planters with highly saturated red, yellow, and orange flowers and/or child-sized wheelbarrows will cultivate active participation. Most children are drawn to anything on wheels and may be inspired to push a wheelbarrow loaded with vegetable and fruit peels, collected from snack time, to the central hub housing the composting bins.

A loop (like its concentric ring counterpart) supports cooperative learning. Movement in the learning garden flows in a clockwise direction (the door being 12 on a clock dial), beginning with the least intensive activity (at 3 o'clock). When the children arrive at the third station (9 o'clock), they have progressed to the most complex learning activity. The loop has a minimum of three activity stations (3 o'clock, 6 o'clock, 9 o'clock), but depending on the number of children using the garden, additional stations with increasing challenges can be designed to accommodate more children. The compost staging hub is accessible from all points, empowering children to use it under their own volition.

Each station has several elements, including adequate seating proximal to planting beds. Because most children will want to water plants,

LEFT Many clever and efficient ways to store garden implements also support learning and movement. A tower can be used to direct children to follow movement and directional patterns and hang watering cans in specific sequences from high to low, and so on.

RIGHT An elevated hose bib makes access easier for seated gardeners or those who have trouble bending over.

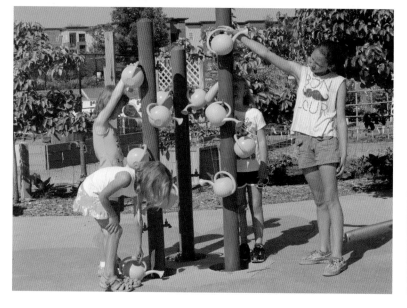

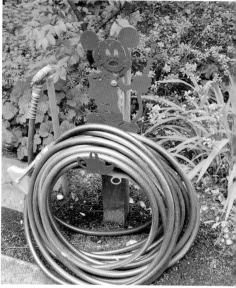

elevated (18 to 24 inches) hose bibs or water faucets are located at each station, offering easy access for seated and standing gardeners. Design clever ways to store child-sized watering cans: on hooks, stacked on poles, or in cubbies. Because some children will be reluctant to engage in the actual gardening task yet need to feel included and part of the group, each station should also contain an alternative learning activity that still supports outdoor learning.

The first station (at 3 o'clock) provides the least intensive opportunities to engage in nature; here, children care for established plantings in a series of at-grade and raised beds, working together and invited to touch, deadhead, and water plants. Children who are less reluctant to get dirty will head for the at-grade beds; those who are more reluctant will likely gravitate to the raised beds. This garden can be planted with sturdy, native seedlings collected from the third station, the growing and harvest space. Learning activities include passively monitoring freestanding drying racks to preserve flowers and leaves for future inspection, or turning a hand-cranked waterwheel for more active engagement.

The second station, the planting station (at 6 o'clock), provides more challenging opportunities. Here children work at mini-potting benches, planting seeds or transplanting seedlings; in time, they will carry individual

More than just fun to operate, turning a waterwheel is a good source of upper body exercise and a way for children to work together to measure water volume.

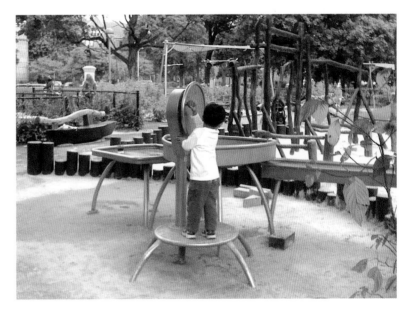

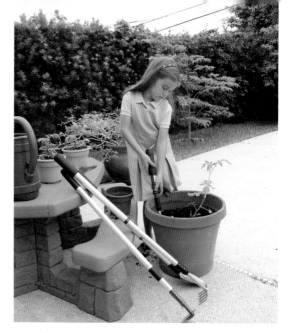

potted plants or push flat carts to the third station. As an alternative to gardening, a multilevel sandbox filled with measuring tools, utensils, sifters, and trucks encourages such concepts as counting, measuring, pouring, and transporting. Design elements include adjustable-height potting benches, some on grass and others on pavement. For some children, standing on grass may be within their comfort level; for others, firm paving is a better option. Storage for ergonomically designed garden tools (like trowels with telescoping handles, for children who cannot or choose not to reach into the planters) should be readily accessible.

Tools with telescoping handles increase the range of opportunities for all gardeners, not just reluctant young ones, to more safely garden from sitting or standing positions.

The third station (at 9 o'clock) is the growing and harvest station, a level, well-drained grassy area. At this point children are becoming more confident, and most can actively tend the plants through their life cycles. Supplied by seedlings germinated in the planting station, the growing and harvest area also requires ample storage to house watering cans and garden tools and tables. In the harvest area, children tend the at-grade and raised beds, cultivating seasonally viable vegetables and herbs, and prepare simple meals with the produce harvested. Alternative learning activities include building blocks and using magnifying glasses, chalk, and chalkboards for inspection and documentation of rocks, plants, or insects. Lean-to shelters and other small wire structures planted with climbing vines or vegetables function as retreats to which children can retire to compile data from their "scientific inquiries."

The surrounding fence should be aesthetically pleasing; think of it as an object of beauty. The eight-foot-high fence deters unwelcome visitors from coming into the garden. When camouflaged with densely planted sunflowers, amaranth, corn, or other tall grains, grasses, bamboos, or fruit trees, the fence becomes a verdant display of seasonal interest. Hanging easy-to-read thermometers in the greenery or on the fence adds an additional layer of learning for children to observe and monitor the weather. Your client and budget will determine the best way to beautify the fence.

In addition to basic mathematical, science, and language concepts, life cycles, sequencing, observation, responsibility, decision-making, cooperation, confidence, and patience are a few of the skills learned in this garden. All are skills that are easily transferrable and applicable to a child's continuing life journey.

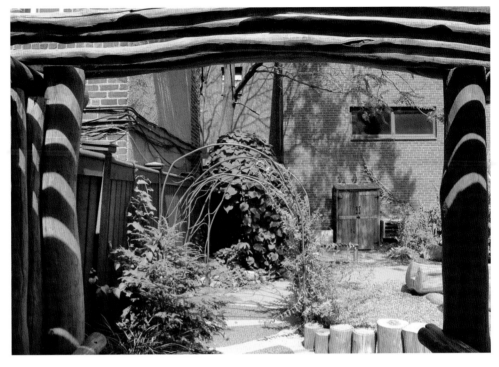

Small vine-covered structures are natural cubicles where children can think and work in relative quiet. This intimate vine tunnel is also a retreat for children who need to be alone to observe rather than participate.

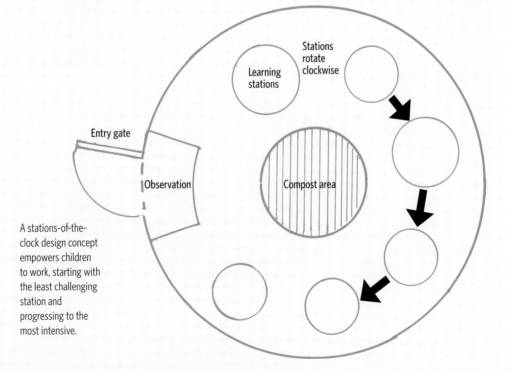

A stations-of-the-clock design concept empowers children to work, starting with the least challenging station and progressing to the most intensive.

CLOSER LOOK

Green Chimneys

Set on over 350 acres in Brewster, New York, Green Chimneys fills an important niche for K–12 students who have been unsuccessful in traditional classroom models. Founded in 1947, the school offers children and young adults with emotional and learning challenges standard educational curricula and adjunct courses such as woodworking and art; but it is most famous for its renowned nature-based programs, which embrace the worth and value of all living things as means to improve functional capacity and reconnect with self and family. On a main-campus school garden and working organic farm, children participate in all aspects of the growing process, from seed to table. The school garden is an integral part of the curriculum, a living lab where children learn language, math, and science concepts; it is also a place for students to learn to navigate interpersonal challenges, as they are teamed up and set off on scavenger hunts to find and identify different types of root crops, squash, or butterflies or other insects. Vegetable teepees, trellises, and planters fill the 900-square-foot outdoor learning space. There are 40 raised beds, border gardens, a berry patch, and, just outside a greenhouse, the tea garden, where perennial herbs are grown and made into teas, or dried and used throughout the winter months in life skills classes. Produce, fruit, and herbs are harvested and served in the cafeteria. During inclement weather, a screened gazebo becomes an alternative classroom. On the organic farm, with staff supervision, students run a vegetable stand and sell honey harvested from beehives and maple syrup tapped from the farm's trees, among other locally grown products. For many, this opportunity to engage in hands-on learning is a highly motivating part of their educational curriculum and a path to future vocational pursuits.

TOP Making lists of fruits and vegetables that contain seeds is the first step in a multipart learning experience where children work together in small teams to locate those same plants in the garden.

BOTTOM Hands-on, experiential learning in the garden is at the heart of the Green Chimneys educational model.

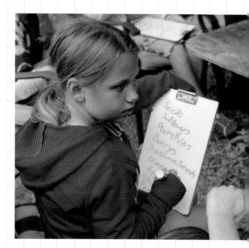

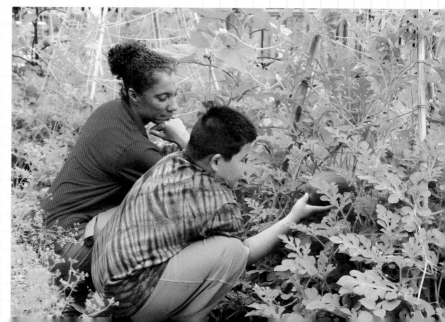

Gardens for Intergenerational Learning

Learning gardens can also link generations around a shared objective, eliciting powerful memories as elder participants share their past and youth dream about their future. They connect and reconnect children with grandparents, parents, and mentors who are or were gardeners, ready to proudly pass on skills learned over a lifetime. With an increasing number of people tasked to raise their grandchildren, such learning gardens can become the common ground to connect multiple generations.

Garden rooms are, once again, a great organizing principle to guide the layout of an intergenerational learning garden. Each room is designed with a different purpose—a kitchen, a reading room, a mad science lab, a history archive—offering prompts for shared activities from which conversations can germinate. Architectural or landscape room dividers can spatially demarcate the spaces and function as natural sound barriers. Each space should have adequate shade and flexible seating options, an accessible bathroom, and drinking fountain.

In the kitchen room, raised planters and garden beds are filled with cutting flowers, herbs, and farm-to-fork vegetables. Planters at differing heights provide choices for young and old to kneel, stand, or sit as they cultivate and harvest the bounty and savor the aromas while cleaning and preparing them for the noontime meal.

In the reading room, furnished with oversized rocking and glider chairs or bench swings, children listen to or read stories, snuggling during these intimate exchanges with their elders. The room should evoke the qualities of softness and dreaminess. Landscape features may include green hedges and subtly colored planters filled with leaves and flowers in muted colors.

The mad science room is furnished with table-height planters overflowing with exotic succulents that inspire gentle touch. Plants with oversized leaves and strangely shaped flowers will spark conversation. Discrete storage for paper, markers, and magnifying glasses facilitates close examination of the plants.

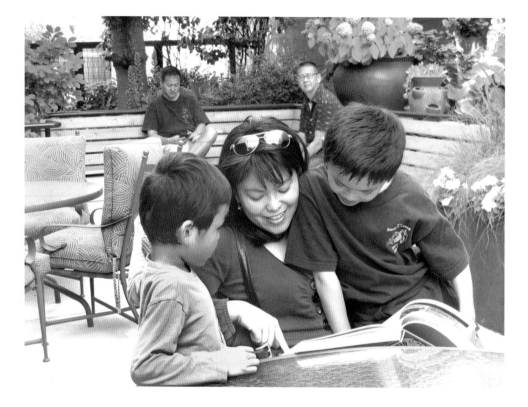

In the history room, mature visitors reminisce with their younger visitors about what gardening means to them. Many pleasant garden memories will center on aromatic herbs. To elicit spontaneous stories, herb gardens filled with medicinal, kitchen, and aromatic herbs to touch and smell should be a central component of this archive. An old clawfoot tub filled with plants is a whimsical prompt for grandparents to share stories about life in the "olden days."

Furnished with ample seating, a garden has the capacity to host intergenerational storytelling and reading.

DESIGN CONSIDERATIONS

Besides children and adults who ambulate on their own, intergenerational learning gardens need to accommodate children (some in strollers), those who need assistance, and those using wheeled mobility devices. Sensory changes, especially declining vision and hearing, often accompany the aging process. To accommodate those with visual impairment, signage and wayfinding prompts should be easily comprehensible and readable.

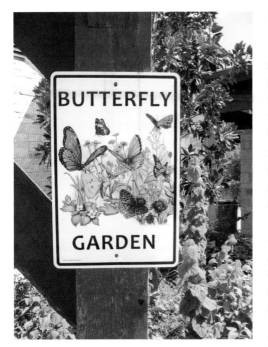

Signage with high contrast between text and background and easily recognizable images increases the garden's usability for all people.

Lettering should be done in a large sans-serif font, in a color that contrasts with the background.

Familiar icons reduce the amount of text needed and increase legibility. Glare from glossy surfaces or bright sun may cause temporary blindness. Gently filtered natural light is ideal for reading signs or safely navigating garden paths. At night, artificial path lighting will increase visibility and use (see chapter 2 for more on lighting options). Shadows cast from pergolas or arbors may be misinterpreted as stairs and should be sited using sun/shadow studies to minimize this effect.

For older adults with hearing impairments, design challenges include the buffering of industrial or other noxious noises. Try to minimize these distractions by using dense vegetation to absorb the sounds without an echo effect, or introducing the ambient sound of gently flowing water. Finally, locate clearly visible and easy-to-use emergency call systems in centralized locations. An intergenerational learning garden needs to balance the physical and sensory needs and constraints of older adults while maintaining engaging opportunities for younger participants; it should be an interesting, versatile place for all ages.

Peace Gardens

Conflict mediation traditionally takes place indoors—in a court of law, classroom, or counselor's office. Therapeutic gardens offer neutral and nonthreatening environments where conflicts involving disparate marginalized groups vying for dominance can be mediated. Gangs often engage in violent acts as initiation rites, or to claim territory or prove their machismo. When provided with planting beds, a place to cultivate or create recreational activities, all participants enter upon a shared endeavor that requires trust and interdependence. These qualities align with principles of mediation and require continued stewardship and acceptance of others.

Some people associate vegetation with crime, assuming that predators may be hiding in the woods behind shrubs or mounds. Research refutes this assumption, showing that green areas surrounding inner-city highrises resulted in lower incidences of aggression, incivility, and violence, and lower rates and fear of crime (Kuo and Sullivan 2001a, 2001b). Siting a reconciliation or mediation garden in nature builds on these beneficial attributes and incorporates the inherent positive properties of plants.

How often have you heard people say so-and-so "never learned how to play in the sandbox"? There is some real truth to that expression. Early in life children engage in parallel play. Using the same space and situated side by side, play evolves into a complex system of shared experiences. As children grow, they learn to express themselves through play, to act out anger, fantasies, frustration, or joy, and to expand their imaginations. Play is that important venue where children learn about themselves, about others, and how to get along. What children learn about relationship-building through early play experiences influences later adult relationships, and the important role that outdoor environments have in nurturing this process is just beginning to be explored. A Canadian study looked at the relationship between green school grounds and social inclusivity; the results were that children who felt isolated based on gender, class, race, or ability felt more accepted on greener school grounds (Dyment and Bell 2008). This suggests that green spaces promote, in a broad sense, social inclusion.

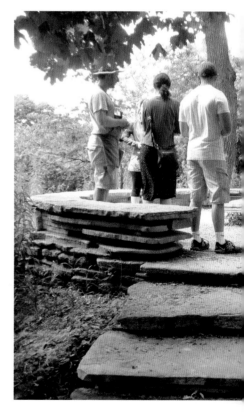

Landscape architect Jens Jensen developed the council ring concept, a meeting or gathering place in nature. This council ring, located in Chicago's Lincoln Park, was designed by Jensen's protégé Alfred Caldwell.

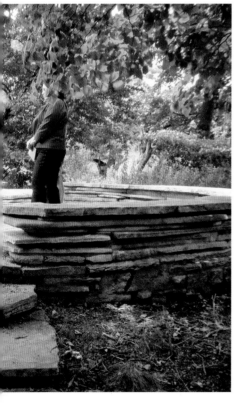

DESIGN CONSIDERATIONS

The most important feature of a peace garden is neutrality. Most gangs have "colors" that signify their membership and allegiance. In White Center, Washington, a place shaped by a recent influx of immigrants from Asia, Latin America, and Africa, a public forum was held to select colors for a rainwater harvesting system in a community garden. Many attendees were attracted to blue (symbolizing water), and it was thought that the bright blue that was chosen would add vibrancy to the community garden and larger park. As the paint was being purchased, a frantic call came from the county project manager, who explained that neither red nor blue could be used, as each represented active gangs. The fear was that one or the other of the gangs would assume possession of the park if either color were used. The cistern was ultimately painted yellow, and the park functions as a place of neutrality. Though both gangs frequent the park, no structures have been tagged, no violent confrontations have been documented, and non-gang community members use the park and community garden without fear or intimidation.

Most mediation gardens have a space where discussions occur. A circular space is ideal, since it is harder to declare or appropriate a side when the space is round. In a circular council ring, participants face each other in directed dialogue to resolve differences, practice respect, and negotiate and dismantle imposed boundaries and animosity.

To minimize any sense of entrapment, keep the garden open on all sides and avoid small, isolated spaces. Maintain clear sightlines and visibility to reduce fear and PTSD triggers. Peace gardens should be balanced, with spaces for passive activities (such as talking and discussion) and for more active programs (such as impromptu baseball games and concerts). In addition to the council ring, a level, well-drained lawn, play courts, walking paths, picnic tables, and sensory and vegetable gardens are necessary therapeutic elements. Participants must not feel threatened; they need to maintain a sense of control, inclusion, choice, and focus. For some users, a strict formality is threatening and triggers memories of prison camps or barracks. For others, this sense of order may increase focus by offering clear legibility and sense of control, a reassuring counterpoint to their highly chaotic lives.

Rainier Beach Urban Farm

Michael Neguse arrived in Seattle in 1984, an Eritrean refugee from Sudan, where, as a guerilla fighter, he had witnessed terrible scenes of death. "I volunteered—I defended my country, my family, and I didn't know what they would ask me to do. It was horrible, but in my country no one talks about it—we hold it in." A low-flying plane buzzed above the garden where he stood on a recent morning. "I hate that sound. It reminds me of home."

After emigrating, he became a crime prevention coordinator at Yesler Terrace, a public housing project in Seattle. His days were productive, his nights racked with nightmares from which he'd awaken drenched in sweat and unable to explain his strange behavior to his wife or children. He discovered that when gardening, his chronic depression and feelings of isolation abated, but most of the green spaces near Yesler had been co-opted by addicts and prostitutes, and residents were fearful to enter them. So Michael recruited other East African immigrants experiencing similar trauma and, in partnership with Seattle Tilth, created the Rainier Beach Urban Farm. He became a community advocate, encouraging other refugees to talk about their past memories and present troubles, and was instrumental in bringing the Refugee Women's Alliance youth program to the farm, where reconciliation between former warring ethnicities is a reality and languages such as Somali, Oromo, Amharic, and Arabic can be heard. Many of the immigrant gardeners had experienced refugee camps and civil wars, and they opened up to Michael, breaking the culturally adopted code of silence and admitting their insecurities, sorrow, and guilt.

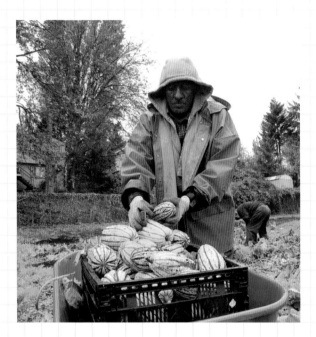

Squash is a staple at the Rainier Beach Urban Farm, where conflict mediation takes place outside and the sense of belonging to a community is strengthened.

The farm is a peaceful refuge, a place where Ethiopian and Eritrean refugees participate in a conciliation project focused on learning practical skills and growing, harvesting, preparing, and consuming healthful

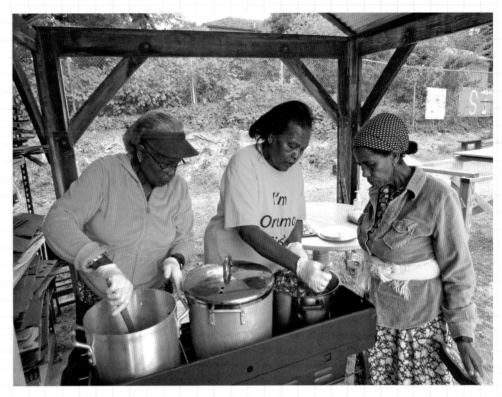

TOP Working side by side and learning from each other, these women, one Eritrean and two Ethiopian, prepare a weekly community lunch from the peace garden's bounty.

BOTTOM The communal meal brings those who have been in conflict together. Around the shared acts of cooking and eating, those who know little about each other explore their commonalities, and the barriers to conciliation are shed.

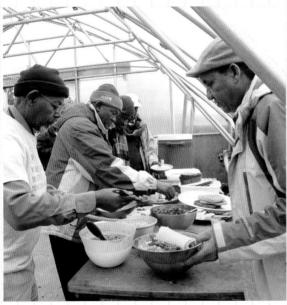

food. Thirteen participants arrive early each morning to hoe, weed, plant, and water their beds. Newcomers are greeted warmly and join in work parties that are repairing the greenhouses, tilling amendments into the soil, and turning the compost. Every Friday, after harvesting squash and chard from the orderly rows of winter greens, or tomatoes and basil from the greenhouses, three women, one Eritrean and two Ethiopian, come together in the kitchen to chop and dice the bounty as they prepare traditional East African dishes on outdoor gas grills. Once served, all gather for lunch around a 40-foot-long table, forging supportive, sustaining friendships between the two ethnicities.

Vocational Training Gardens

Vocational training gardens serve marginalized groups, including the homeless, veterans, adults with developmental disabilities or mental health issues. Participants learn about cultivating plants and growing a microbusiness, perhaps selling their produce at local grocers, supplying restaurants, or even making and distributing salsa. Vocational training gardens are purposeful and mission-driven, inspiring participants to get up in the morning and go to work in the garden. Because so much more than learning about plants occurs, vocational training gardens are well suited for homeless shelters, veterans hospitals or clinics, outpatient programs, and adult day training centers.

On the outskirts of Jacksonville, Florida, veterans participate in a six-month fellowship training program in farming techniques at Veterans Farm, founded and directed by Purple Heart recipient Adam Burke. The farm specializes in blueberries and peppers, and the public is welcome

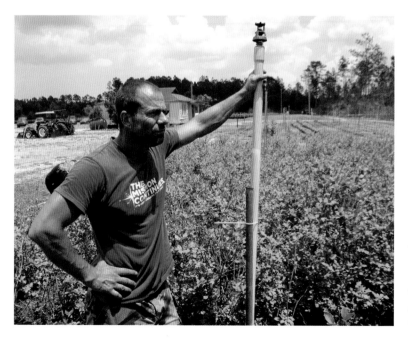

A trainee farmer pauses and reflects for a moment. In-ground blueberries in this area of the farm are dug up and sold to waiting customers.

to come and pick fruit and purchase pepper plants and jam made from the farm's berries. The design is accessible; most of the more than 4,500 blueberry bushes are in pots, and the rows between all the pots and plants are wide enough to accommodate wheeled mobility devices, making it possible for everyone who wants to farm to learn how. The farm is a safe place for veterans to learn important vocational and interpersonal skills, regain a sense of hope and purpose, and to reconnect with themselves through a connection with the land.

DESIGN CONSIDERATIONS

Vocational training gardens need barrier-free workspaces and growing beds that enable wheeled mobility users to access plants straight on, avoiding painful twisting movements. Users will have a wide range of cognitive, physical, and psychological abilities. Some will have mobility challenges or difficulty using their hands and arms. Others will be physically weak, emotionally fragile, or learn more slowly than their peers, and some individuals will seek refuge when coping becomes difficult. Ample shade will accommodate gardeners whose medications increase photosensitivity. Fatigue levels will vary, and places for rest and seating should be sited nearby. These are both productive and social gardens, places for trainees to learn from and support each other. Gathering spaces need to be flexible, uplifting, and facilitate social connections; they are where participants will eat, share tips, discuss the day's activities—all much-needed counterpoints to the isolation many experience. The garden needs to be focused and goal-oriented. There needs to be clear delineation of responsibilities and, in some cases, contracts that participants abide by, to ensure that the garden runs smoothly.

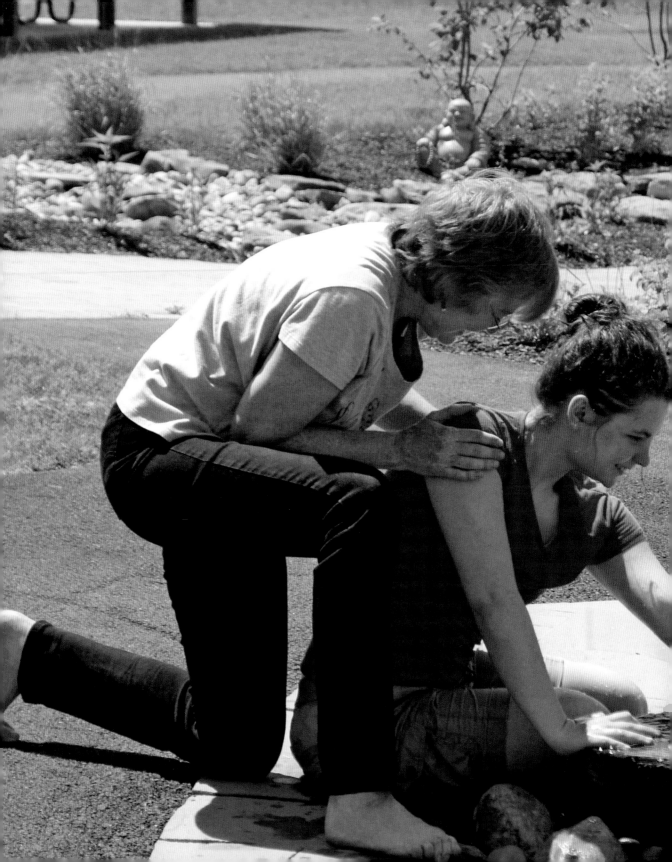

CHAPTER SIX
SENSORY GARDENS

Providing all people, those with and those without disability or disease, abundant opportunities to nourish their sensory systems in well-designed therapeutic gardens is important because everything in our daily lives is guided by the senses. For those whose sensory systems are altered due to neurological conditions, disease, trauma, or age, response to sensory experiences can be very powerful, sometimes positively and sometimes not. Sensory gardens are typically created for children with autism spectrum disorder (ASD), people undergoing cancer or HIV/AIDS treatment, veterans with PTSD, and those with dementia or other memory loss issues. Designing sensory gardens within botanic gardens is a growing sector of practice for landscape architects.

Depending on whom the design is intended to serve, therapeutic sensory gardens take on different forms and complexity. The challenge is to understand the range of needs and responses of specific users. As always, a collaborative design process brings multiple viewpoints and expertise to better understand, distill, and meet the special needs of all concerned. Sensory gardens are best designed in close collaboration with an occupational therapist with expertise in sensory integration and environmental modification. The collaborative design model creates opportunities for people to do what they want and need to do in nourishing sensory environments.

Shared by Stephanie Murphy: My son Lincoln loves nature. He craves it. When Lincoln was 11 years old he had a hemispherectomy, an invasive brain surgery designed to end the epilepsy that was controlling his life. After the surgery Lincoln spent several weeks in a cramped room in one of New York City's finest hospitals. If you know anything about New York, you know that there is just no space, and this goes double for hospitals. My son is a country boy. He loves the air, wide-open spaces, the sounds of birds, and the feel of grass beneath his bare feet. Is it any wonder that his first request upon arriving home in upstate New York was to take a walk to our lake? This lake is a half a mile into the woods, hidden from humans but home to a dense community of white tail deer, beavers, geese, ducks, a barred owl who glides silently overhead, and sundry fish who seem to linger in the sunny spots of the nearby stream. Despite my fear, Lincoln made it, and much to this mother's delight, he continued to make the trip, sometimes twice or three times a day. Each time he reached the lake, exhaustion would engulf him, and I would help him to lie down on a soft blanket in a sunny patch of warmed pine needles. There he'd sleep and recharge as the owl watched protectively from his perch and the bass and sunfish swam laps nearby him. And while he finally slept deeply, uninterrupted by the beeps and buzzers and constant sensory assault of the hospital, this mother would finally breathe deeply, and begin to relax, allowing the birds, the sun, the breeze, and the sound of her son's rhythmic breathing to heal her, too.

Sensation

Sensory experiences in the garden can be uplifting or relaxing.

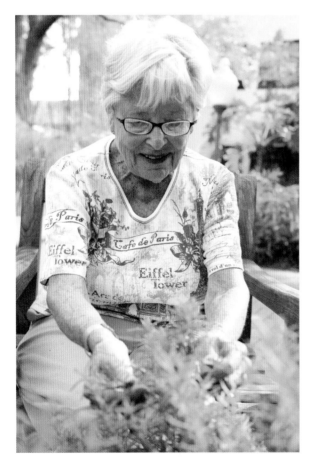

We all know about the five basic senses—touch, taste, smell, sight, and hearing—and sensory gardens usually nourish them all. But there are other sensory systems: kinesthetic, proprioceptive, vestibular, and tactile. Kinesthesia and proprioception help us understand body/spatial relationships and to use exactly the right amount of physical effort to accomplish a task; when people struggle with proprioception and kinesthesia, things like grasping an empty paper cup without crushing it, sitting down on a chair without falling off, or going through a doorway without banging into the frame are challenging. The vestibular system plays a significant role in balance and movement and helps control dizziness. People with overactive vestibular systems tend to get carsick easily and avoid carnival rides and/or boats; people with underactive vestibular systems tend to enjoy swinging and spinning in excess. The tactile system pertains to and crosses over from the basic sense of touch. People with tactile defensiveness interpret touch negatively: a pat on the back feels like a beating, a shirt collar tag feels like needles, touching slimy things feels awful, and getting jostled is too much to cope with.

Think about the relationship between gardens and movement, balance, and touch. You need to know how to design gardens to avoid under- or overstimulation of these foundational sensory systems. We used the word "nourish" (rather than "stimulate") in the first sentence of this chapter and feel it best describes how sensory garden design should work, as for some, stimulation is not appropriate. Sensory garden design is a delicate dance between partners to create the right nourishing outdoor environment for these vulnerable user groups.

Sensory Integration

When our sensory systems are integrated, they help us understand the world. Sensory integration is a normal neurological process that starts in the womb and continues throughout life. Sensory or sensation refers to incoming information from the environment and our bodies. Sometimes we are aware of sensation, such as the sweet perfume of a rose. Other times, we know the exact right amount of pressure to apply with our fingers, hand, and arm to pluck a single juicy ripe raspberry off a vine. Integration is how we interpret (in the brain) and use sensory information. To most of us, the rose smells divine, and its scent makes us feel happy. We are able to pluck the fragile raspberry without taking the branch with it. Intact sensory integration enables us to more or less effortlessly go about our daily lives. For more on sensory integration, see Ayres (2005).

Serious and persistent problems with sensory integration may lead to a diagnosis of sensory processing disorder (SPD), which entails extreme difficulty taking in, processing, and appropriately responding to sensory information. Tactile defensiveness and proprioceptive and vestibular issues are associated with the disorganized nervous system of people with SPD. Children are most frequently diagnosed with SPD, but increasingly adults are receiving the diagnosis. The diagnosis is typically made by occupational therapists trained and certified to administer a standardized assessment, the Sensory Integration and Praxis Test. The impact of SPD can be devastating. Those with SPD often have trouble with relationships, organization, focus, and taking care of themselves. Life is hard. Finding the acceptable balance to manage their sensory challenges is a daily struggle. Well-intentioned design lacking in authentic understanding of SPD significantly diminishes the chances a sensory garden will meet user needs.

At the Leg Up Farm, a nonprofit therapy center for children with disabilities and developmental delays, staff embrace the health benefits of being in nature as a means of sensory enrichment and well-being. Its unique holistic and inclusive model, practiced by educators and occupational, physical, and speech therapists, is based on the idea that life extends beyond the walls of a therapy clinic or classroom. Located on 18 acres in York County, Pennsylvania, this collaboratively designed, sensory-rich campus offers clients, staff, and families a multitude of opportunities to participate in therapy and simultaneously be immersed in nature via

Providing ample opportunities to touch, feel, taste, smell, see, hear, and move is a primary goal of sensory garden design.

universally accessible paths in and out of the woods, a rambling play structure, gardens, horseback riding, and water features—all designed with the idea that they will benefit the children. The outdoor spaces are well used, no matter the season. Cumulatively, they all support the goal of achieving optimal outcomes for clients and their families.

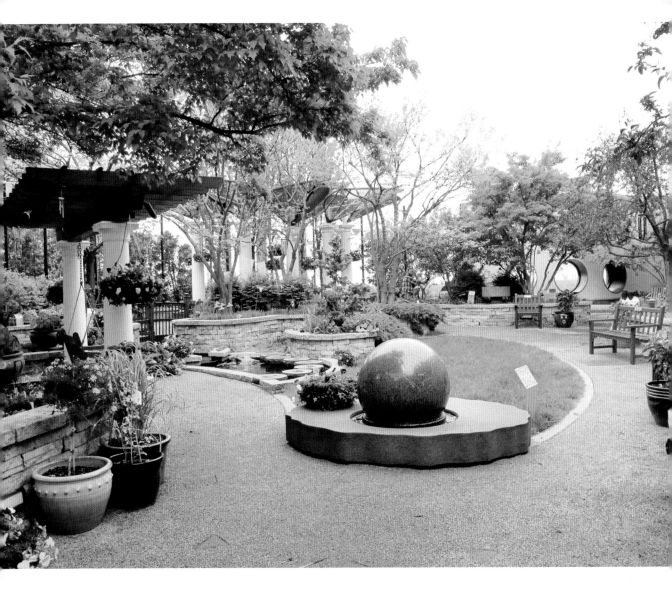

CLOSER LOOK

Dolphin House

To better engage children, clinicians, care staff, and families, Westley Design worked with the Royal Cornwall Hospital Trust (RCHT) to develop a sensory play area at the Dolphin House, a child development center in Truro for preschoolers with complex needs and disabilities. At a series of design workshops, the team from Westley Design asked psychologists, occupational therapists, teaching/care staff, and the children themselves to describe their play experiences, as participants and observers, in the existing challengingly small courtyard. The conversation continued, as the client group visited the workshops of a team of designer/makers, contractors, and artists, to see models and comment on work in progress. This collaboration optimized the functionality and efficiency of the space and created a sense of shared ownership among the stakeholders. The results can be seen in a single, playful piece of sculpture that functions as a focal point in the courtyard, dividing the surrounding spaces into subnodes of varied character and self-directed play and learning opportunities. Clinical and educational staff can select from a range of sensory elements to tailor a creative and appropriate experience for each child.

The central active play structure offers a variety of child-friendly kinesthetic, proprioceptive, and tactile activities that include balancing, sliding, climbing, swinging, and spinning. Container planting allows children to engage in therapeutic gardening activities from standing or sitting positions; the containers are filled with seasonally relevant plantings with sensory appeal, and the children tend them using an array of garden tools that are easy for them to use. Sand and water splash features offer rich and constructional sensory play opportunities. Children engage

OPPOSITE A zero-threshold sandbox enables all children to play equally under the nurturing watch of their teachers and therapists. It is also an opportunity for social gathering, a place for children to learn the important rules of negotiation.

Sand and water elements are adjacent to each other. A shade sail provides protection from the sun and prevents sand from becoming too hot in the summer months.

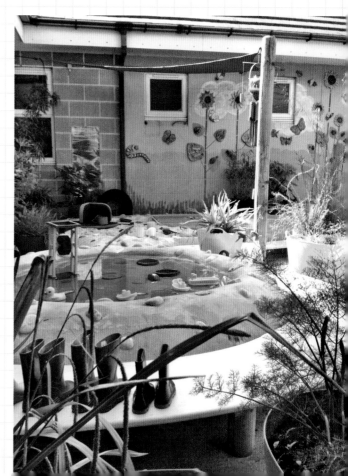

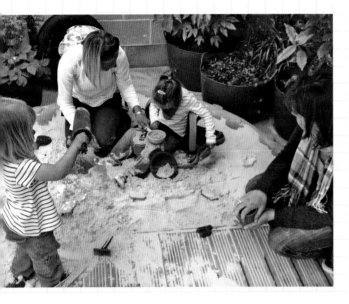

in spontaneous science and math lessons involving measurement and estimating even as they enjoy the tactile experiences that sand and water provide; they build strength and enhance proprioception and kinesthesia by filling and carrying buckets of sand and water from one location to another, while trying to not spill a drop. While designed for play, all these activities are an integral part of the children's therapy programming.

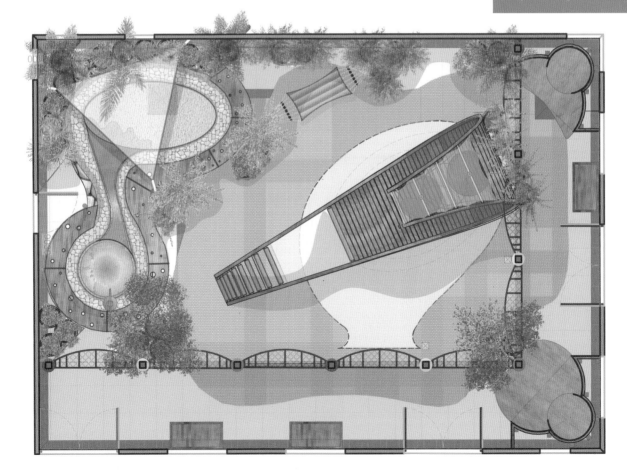

A rendering of the Dolphin House garden.

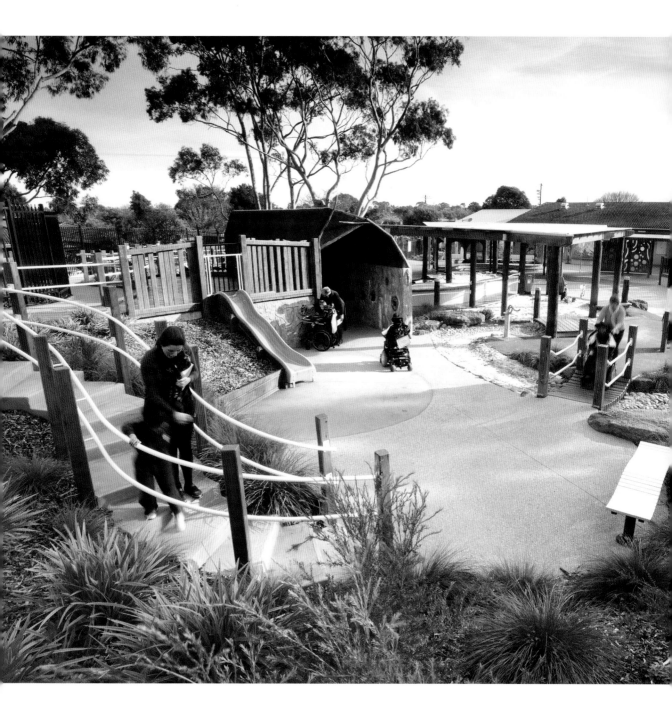

Gardens for Children with ASD

Children with ASD have myriad physical, cognitive, and emotional challenges. As of 2014, the Centers for Disease Control and Prevention found that one in 68 children in the United States has autism (Baio 2014). It is almost five times more common in boys than girls. There is no cure for ASD. Many children (and adults) with ASD, whether diagnosed or not, will also have sensory processing challenges. Current research literature suggests that having access to nature remains beneficial even for children with ASD. Nature, for those with ASD, means sensory environments that nourish and enrich rather than under- or overstimulate. Life can be overwhelming for some children with ASD because their sensory systems are poorly integrated. Many have under- or overresponsive sensory systems. They might not react in the same way as their typically developing peers to sounds, textures, tastes, smells, and visual and movement stimuli. They may cover their ears when hearing birds sing, refuse to touch flower petals, or gaze with unwavering focus on running water. They may

LEFT Walking or rolling over a suspension bridge offers a range of proprioceptive, kinesthetic, and vestibular challenges.

RIGHT Occupational, speech, and physical therapists knowledgeable about sensory integration are an important part of a design team, ensuring that sensory elements provide the appropriate balance between under- and overstimulation.

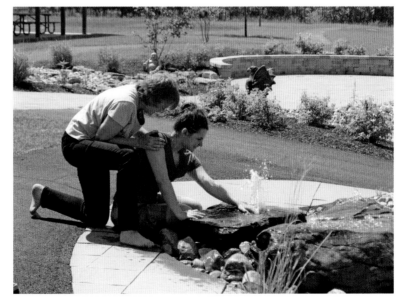

want to swing for hours or refuse to climb a ladder or go down a slide. Many children with ASD also struggle with being flexible and thrive on predictability and routine. It is essential that a child with ASD maintains a feeling of being in control in the sensory garden. The design team's challenge is to find the optimal balance between under- and overstimulation and directed and self-directed opportunities, and to overcome a child's reluctance to participate. For more on autism, visit autismspeaks.org.

DESIGN CONSIDERATIONS

Choose a sensory garden location that is quiet, with the fewest distractions possible. If the site is not naturally screened, architectural or vegetated buffering can diminish extraneous distractions. Circular, curvilinear shapes are well suited to weave through multiple sensory areas: the flow they create through the space is helpful to those with space perception challenges. Open sightlines reduce confusion and disorientation, and curved paths evoke a more relaxed ambience. Avoid toxic plants and plants with thorns or noxious or heady smells, in this or any kind of therapeutic garden.

Surprises and inconsistency can create or elevate anxiety for children with ASD. Signage should replicate simple icons that are consistent with any pictorial communication system used where you are designing the

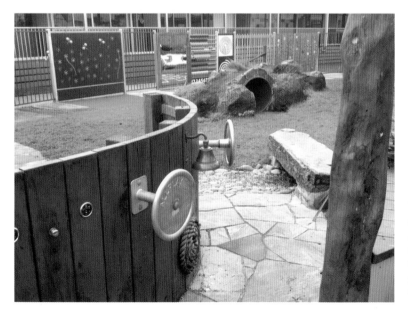

It is necessary to provide spaces both for active engagement and for retreat in a sensory garden, especially at sites where children with sensory issues will be the primary users.

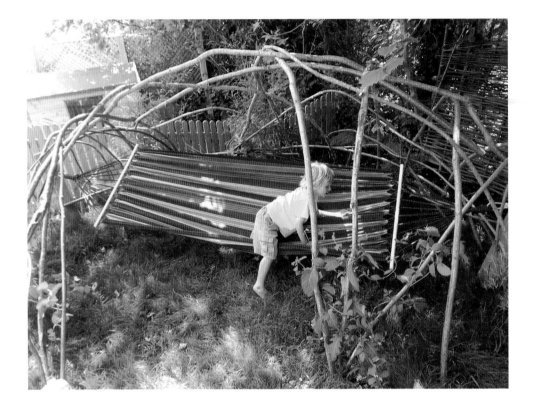

A hammock and enclosed space doubles the chance for soothing decompression. Being in hideaways gives children who feel overwhelmed the chance to collect themselves and prepare for the next moment in the garden.

sensory garden. Place signage at the same height and at similar increments throughout the garden. Predictability and familiarity are important. For example, changing plantings with the seasons or even during the same season may cause distress. Transitioning from one activity to another often makes children with ASD anxious; use gentle transitions from one space in the garden to the next, with "chill" spaces in between for children to rest and reorient themselves before moving on.

Extraneous noise that you may find merely distracting—air conditioning compressor pumps or trees planted so close together that they make scratching and creaking noises when their branches contact the building or each other—may be viscerally disturbing for those with ASD. Avoid plants that make sounds that might scare the user, such as poplar tree leaves that crackle and click. Echoing spaces may be overwhelming and aversive. Be aware that many children with ASD tend to self-stimulate (e.g., rock on toes, twirl, or flap their hands), so it is advisable to avoid wind chimes and kinetic sculpture, which may increase self-stimulatory actions. Like gazing at water, the repetitive motion of the sculpture and chimes may be overly mesmerizing and transfixing.

All water features require forethought. Their auditory characteristics may sound, to a child who is hypersensitive to sound, like industrial dishwashers, in which case quiet water may be a more thoughtful response. Some children with ASD will want to watch running water or let it run over their hands for long periods of time. Others may all but want to climb in it; our friend Susan Sorensen, a retired special education teacher, fondly recalled the enthusiastic reaction of one of her students with ASD to a large water fountain in a sensory garden: "It was like he had just baptized himself with all his clothes on."

People with ASD tend to be photosensitive. Install shade structures at doorways so eyes can slowly adjust to the change in light before venturing into or out from the garden. Provide large areas of shade using trees or covered shelters. Avoid shiny surfaces and elements that reflect light and cause glare such as metallic trashcans, planters, walls, and seating. Those with ASD are likely to look in a single plane instead of scanning the horizon as they move. Colors and materials marking curbs, transitions, and railings provide visual and tactile cueing of pathway boundaries.

Many activities and garden elements might trigger adverse responses in children with ASD, but they need things to do and places to be in that are well designed and appropriate to meet their unique needs. Natural elements such as boulders and logs and some raised beds can be adapted for play or use by staff and children. Suspension bridges, stepping stones, bouncy seats, and climbing elements may enhance body awareness and movement. Some children with ASD will enjoy these elements, and some will find them frightening or overstimulating. Rocking chairs and gliders may be appropriate, as will chairs with armrests; all support body awareness and movement senses. Hammocks, suspended tires, basket swings, and other types of swings that snugly hug and wrap around the body may also improve body awareness and be soothing for some children with ASD. Providing options is important.

Resilient ADA playground matting is a good impact-resistant surfacing, but it can be challenging for some children with ASD because the bounciness of the matting may disrupt their balance. Be judicious and if possible, locate it only beneath climbing and movement elements. Alternatively you may select rubberized tiles that cushion falls and avoid

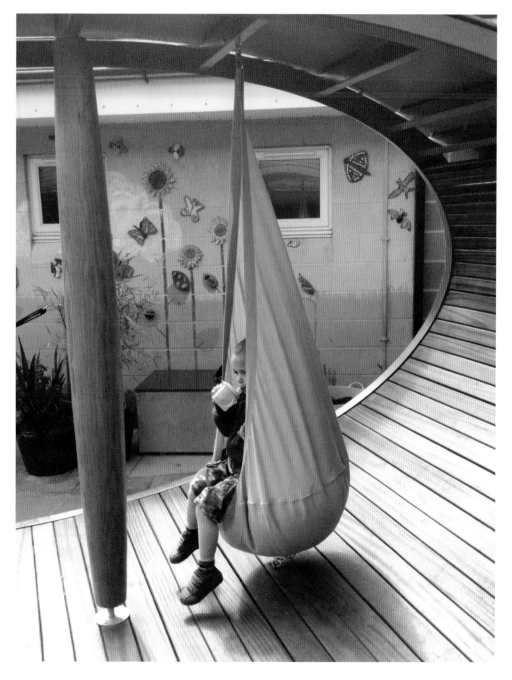

Swings that envelop the body tightly may feel good to some children with ASD: they find it comforting because it provides substantial body awareness cues.

abrasions, but are more stable than resilient matting. Design soothing nook areas, small willow branch tunnels, and nests and valleys of soft grass for children to hide in and collect and reorient themselves when they feel overwhelmed or when approaching a transition in the garden. Site a nook near the entrance to the garden, as it is the biggest transition. Temple Grandin, a professor of animal science at Colorado State University and a world-renowned expert on animal welfare, has autism. Based on her work with livestock animals, she designed a "self-squeeze" machine to use when feeling overwhelmed. Tunnels, nests, and valleys can achieve similar outcomes.

Bamboo, soft ornamental grasses, and smooth boulders encourage and tolerate intensive touching. Mosaics, brick, or exterior terrazzo may also have appealing tactile qualities. Pathway surfaces that make noise like crushed gravel or shells, or feel uncomfortable on hypersensitive feet are not recommended. Avoid prickly grass. It is entirely possible that you will not have many grassy areas in this type of sensory garden. Ground-level or standing-height pots containing soil, sand, or other tactile materials allow children to explore them on their own terms. Large bowls of palm-sized river rocks or smooth shells along a central path enable children to calm and soothe themselves by holding or rubbing the objects in their hands.

It is impossible to isolate sensory experiences. Unless you are blind, you cannot just smell and touch a plant, you also see it. To design for the senses, use movement and balance elements as anchors for the garden and strategically place nook spaces, swings, and seating between them and/or adjacent to suspension bridges or climbing zones, so children can choose the activities that they need. In each of these areas select swaths of similarly colored plants. Plants with flowers or foliage in warm yellows, reds, and oranges may be planted in the stepping stones area. Rich green,

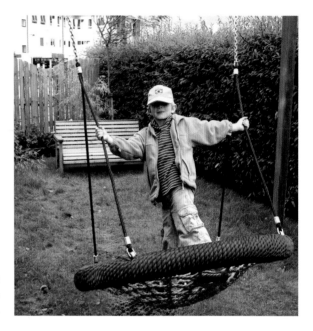

One swing that provides options to sit, stand, or lie flat is a good choice for a sensory garden.

smooth-textured succulents may be planted in the climbing area. Tree bark and leaves with a slightly sticky texture (like those of rosemary and lavender) might be featured in the bridge area. Lavender has a soothing fragrance as well, but some children with tactile challenges may have a negative response when they touch (or smell) it, so alternative aromatic plantings with softer and less-textured leaves may be selected.

Some children may find the bridge area too challenging and instead gravitate to the climbing area. Some may enjoy the sticky leaves, while others move to the nooks or water feature. While you want to avoid plants and hardscape that may amplify negative sensory responses, you want to encourage children to reach beyond their limits, albeit at their pace and on their terms, so offer them choices. Sensory garden design for children with ASD involves significant research, understanding, forethought, and intensive collaboration.

LEFT Sensory elements that connect water with textural elements and novel access address multiple sensory systems simultaneously.

RIGHT To ascend or descend a rope ladder requires integration of the visual, tactile, vestibular, kinesthetic, and proprioceptive senses.

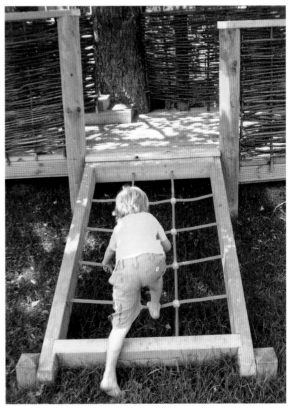

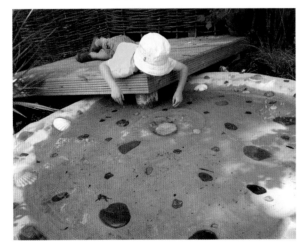

CLOSER LOOK

Carter School

Boston's William E. Carter School is a public school for children (up to age seven years 11 months) with profound developmental delays. Its 0.4-acre sensory garden was designed by David Berarducci Landscape Architecture (based on a conceptual design by Martha Tyson and in close collaboration with Carter School parents and staff) as an oasis for learning and exploration that specifically meets the needs of students. All surfaces are level and easily navigable, and children, all of whom are either in wheelchairs or require assistance with ambulation, can access the garden directly from their classrooms via electronic doors. Once in the garden they follow a wide figure-8 path with color contrast edging. Tall ornamental grasses line a curving secondary path; as students journey along it, they can feel the leaves and feathery flowering stalks touch

Level paths with color contrast edging for students with visual challenges lead to a series of destinations in the garden.

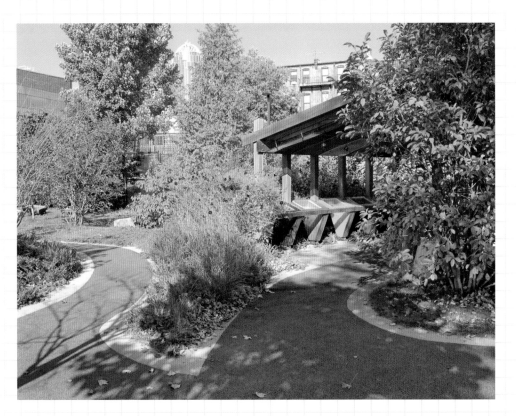

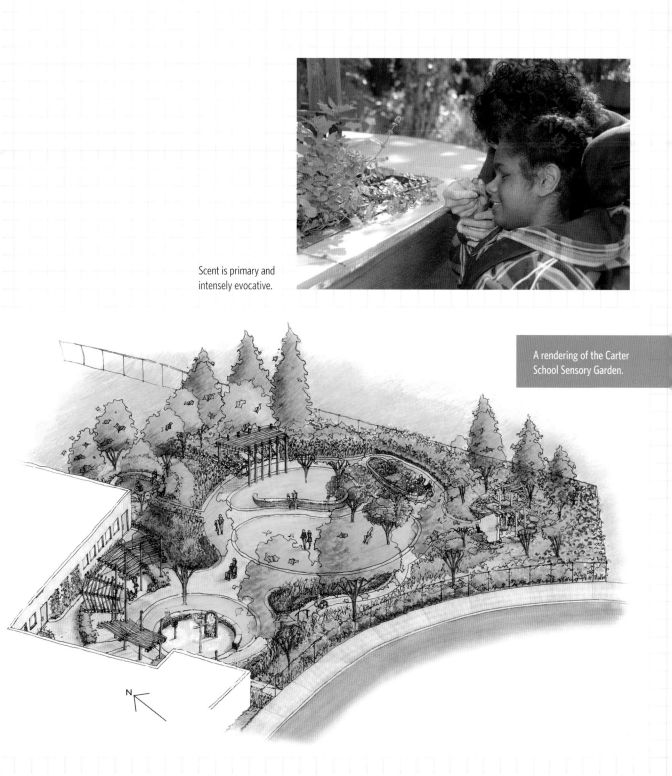

Scent is primary and intensely evocative.

A rendering of the Carter School Sensory Garden.

N

CLOSER LOOK: CARTER SCHOOL *(continued)*

their hands and faces. Side paths lead to a swing area with large molded seats with safety belts and a wheelchair platform. Graceful magnolia and weeping cherry trees provide shade and visual interest; flowering vines cover three pergolas, under which are tables. These and other quiet areas off the main path are ideal spots to relax and eat, observe the activities in the garden, or work with a teacher or therapist.

Wheelchair-height switches that students can activate with their hands, arms, or elbows control various water features; these are an ongoing source of delight and wonder for the children, especially on warm days when, for example, a soothing mist wafts off a pergola's roof. Wheelchairs can easily roll up to and under an elevated planter that allows students to work together to plant, weed, and harvest produce.

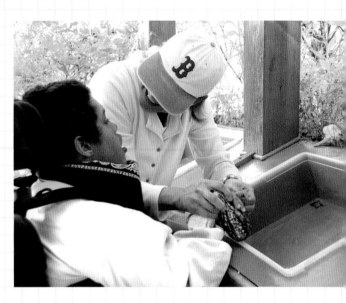

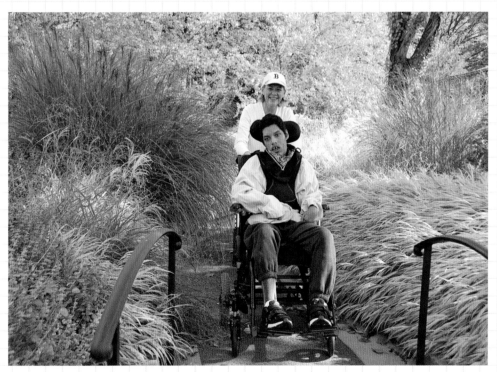

TOP Angled to provide easy wheelchair accessibility, each sorting bin holds a sensory element for children to explore. Something as simple as an ornamental gourd provides several tactile experiences: smooth, rough, cool, bumpy, and dry.

BOTTOM Ornamental grasses are both visually and texturally appealing. Railings dot this path, making it an ideal place to practice ambulation skills.

Wheelchair-accessible bins that can be filled with items such as sand, water, and other tactile objects are used for sensory play and therapy. Aromatic herbs are massed together and invite being touched and sniffed by children who are passing by. A central focal point is a large silver ball, which spins and provides children who sit upon it with a panoramic view of the garden. At the Carter School, education and therapy have moved from the classroom into a place of beauty, tranquility, and sensory enrichment.

A wheelchair-height touch switch operates the water feature in this quiet circular nook.

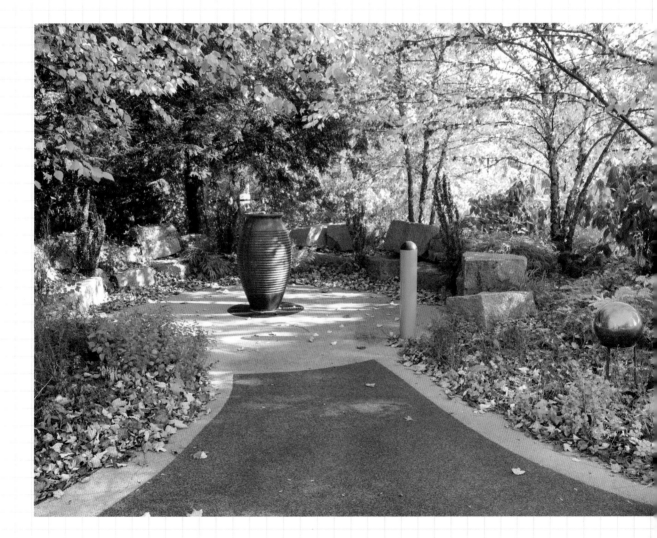

Gardens for Treatment Centers

To design a purposeful sensory garden for people who are being treated for or recovering from illness, one must understand their needs, preferences, and challenges. For example, it is tempting to infuse a sensory garden for cancer or HIV/AIDS treatment centers with aromatic herbs and flowers, but people undergoing chemotherapy often have aversive responses to scents, even to those that may have been appealing in the past. Avoid, therefore, including strongly fragrant plants, or devote a discrete section of the garden to them, one that can be bypassed by patients who respond negatively to them. Listen to your clients and focus on creating uplifting and joyful visual appeal; many of the individuals who will be using the garden will have experienced sensory deprivation while receiving medical treatment. Certain colors, especially very aggressive ones such as cadmium red or yellow, may be inappropriate for some people receiving cancer care, as they are reminiscent of blood or other bodily fluids.

Near and distant views over an expansive body of water with a gently spouting fountain focal point—all enhance a garden's sensory appeal.

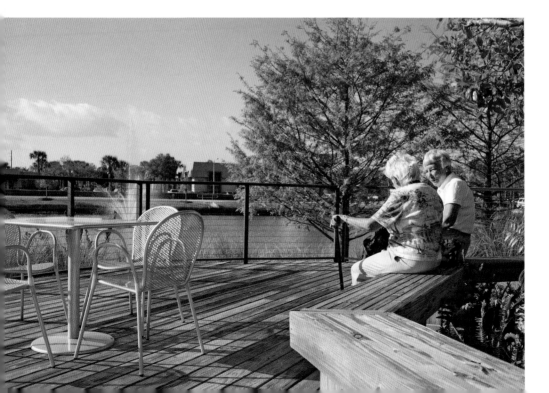

DESIGN CONSIDERATIONS

Create auditory experiences and near and distant soft views within the garden to foster restoration, resilience, and improved sense of control. An abundance of nearby rich plantings surrounding key overlooks to more distant features or winding paths leading to lush destinations provide much-needed visual redirection, mystery, and positive distraction.

An unpublished research study completed at the Jacqueline Fiske Garden of Hope showed that a sense of hopefulness during or following cancer treatment was highest for those who participated in directed social

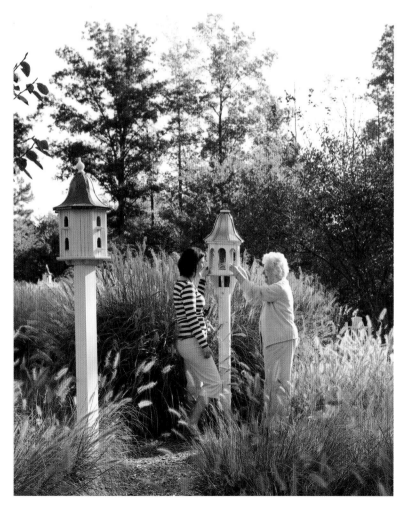

Positive distractions like filling bird feeders may decrease the anxiety that invariably accompanies medical treatment.

horticulture activities in a garden, as compared to those who attended a motivational support group in a windowless room, or a group who walked in the garden and did reflective journaling. Participants felt optimistic and at peace while outside in the garden, working hands-on with plant-related materials; it shifted their focus to the present.

Sounds should be muted. Evocative rain chains suspended over rain barrels are visually appealing and emit gentle sound while demonstrating environmental sensitivity and sustainability. Rustling tree branches (where appropriate) and waving grasses are more universally appealing than clanking wind chimes. Musical preference is highly personal, so piped-in music can be problematic. Better that those who want to listen to music do so on an increasingly affordable, portable personal music device, with earphones.

DESIGN CONTRAINDICATIONS

A common side effect of chemotherapy is damage to the peripheral nervous system; the resulting peripheral neuropathy impairs sensation to the arms and legs, causing symptoms such as numbness, tingling, and burning. Balance and body awareness can be impacted by peripheral neuropathy. Fatigue is also a common side effect of chemotherapy and radiation. To accommodate these side effects, paths should be smooth, level, and bordered with raised edging and hand railings. Avoid plantings that are sharp or have thorns or other hazardous qualities. Rocking motions can increase nausea, another common side effect of chemotherapy, and the rockers on a rocking chair often extend beyond the frame of the chair, posing a tripping hazard for those with peripheral neuropathy (and dementia). For both reasons, don't use rocking chairs in therapeutic gardens at cancer treatment centers. Provide more stable seating options. Reconsider any wooden seating, or if it is used, sand and apply exterior marine varnish or high-quality paint to reduce the risk of splinters; synthetic wood, exterior fabrics, or stone slabs (if the climate is not too cold) are better alternatives. Shiny metal absorbs heat, causes glare, and can burn already highly sensitive skin; it should not be used for seating or planters.

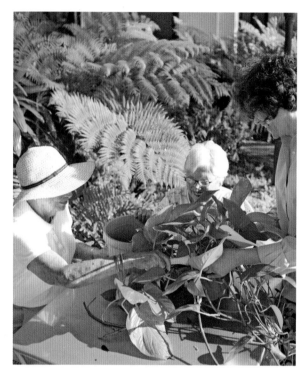

The benefits of an occupational therapy session are heightened in a sensory garden.

Gardens for Veterans with PTSD

Many military personnel returning from recent combat have polytrauma, major physical as well as emotional wounds. Post-traumatic stress disorder is triggered by exposure to a terrifying experience (stressor); responses to that stressor range from helplessness and hyperanxiety to intense fear or horror. Symptoms associated with PTSD are intrusive recollection, avoidant/numbing, and hyperarousal. Sensory gardens for veterans with PTSD, usually located at VA hospitals and clinics, military installations, or memorial sites, must be defensible spaces: for veterans or anyone with PTSD, the fear of recurring trauma is real. For more on PTSD, visit ptsd.va.gov.

Covered spaces off a path provide the scaffolding for social activity and re-engagement with self and others.

DESIGN CONSIDERATIONS

Avoid locating the sensory garden in an area with low visibility. Sightlines must be clear and entries and exits visible from all points in the garden. There should be no perceived spaces from which a (figurative) attacker might lurk. Gardens that are readily perceived as a whole will be more comfortable than those that are compartmentalized. If the garden has "rooms," they need clearly defined containment and means to ensure that someone cannot hide in or approach from behind. These gardens must contain no sharp turns, blind corners, or plantings that obscure paths. Wayfinding needs to be clear and unambiguous. Loud noises can be very disturbing for those with PTSD. Avoid plantings whose sounds and appearance overwhelm the space; they may compound the symptoms of PTSD. Vegetated buffers that can absorb sound, especially when the garden abuts parking lots or busy streets, are recommended.

Choosing outdoor elements that address the symptoms of PTSD is challenging. Consider water features, bird feeders, immersive plantings that support fascination and coherence, and representational art, but avoid the color red in all elements, as it is associated

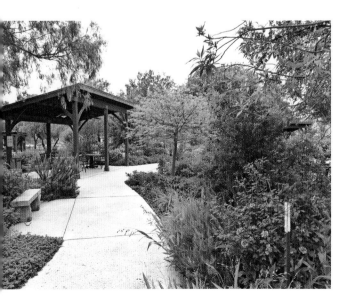

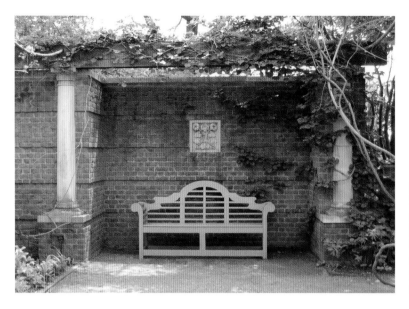

Sensory gardens for those with PTSD require that rooms be designed so there is no potential for someone to approach from or hide behind the space.

with anger and aggressive thoughts. Include distant views of peaceful nature and flexible space for multiple and diverse activities; both elements are positive distractions from intrusive recollections, ways to redirect thoughts. Easy-to-read plant identification signs, a bulletin board for announcements, walkways of differing surfaces, sensory-enrichment opportunities, and small social spaces are important to address avoidant/numbing symptoms; all support re-engagement and reconnection with oneself or others. Elements to tamp down hyperarousal symptoms may include picnic and barbeque spaces, separated smoking areas, glider and rocking chairs, meditative opportunities, and soothing sounds; all promote relaxation.

To accommodate veterans and their families, including infrastructure for meaningful and purposeful activities such as rehabilitation and horticultural therapies, exercise, recreation, and vocational pursuits may amplify the garden's beneficial effects. While some veterans will choose to come to this sensory garden to reflect and journal or read, many will desire activities like sports, physical conditioning, socializing, celebrations, and barbeques. Linking a sensory experience to exercise and cooking can be achieved by installing wheelchair-friendly raised beds with culinary herbs in proximity to the outdoor kitchen. An outdoor kitchen should be universally designed to accommodate standing and seated grilling. Sensory experiences are important, but for veterans with PTSD, they may be the background rather than the focus of this garden. The sensory elements should frame the garden but not necessarily define it.

Gardens for People with Dementia

According to Alzheimer's Disease International (2010), an estimated 115.4 million people will be living with some form of dementia or memory loss by 2050. For those with dementia, an appealing and meaningful destination is a sensory garden. Nursing home administrators have noted that many residents who are confused and agitated when inside are transformed once outside; restlessness significantly diminishes, and mood almost always improves. A caveat: some users become more agitated and want to leave the facility altogether when they have a view of the world beyond. Besides serving memory care nursing facilities, sensory gardens also belong at adult day care centers.

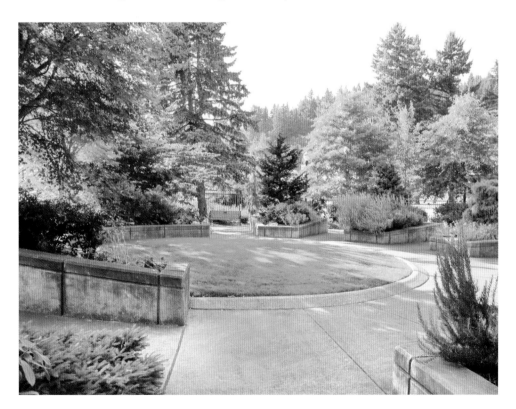

If contained on all sides and with sightlines from all points, those with dementia or other memory issues can wander through a garden on their own.

DESIGN CONSIDERATIONS

Memory care facilities are often designed to look and function as much as possible like domestic environments, while still operating under a medical model. This homelike design approach helps those with Alzheimer's disease and other forms of dementia remain oriented to their surroundings for as long as possible. The sensory garden will ideally be an extension of the homelike environment; it must be located within a safe and protected area, clearly visible from the nurse's station or other indoor supervisory vantage point. A courtyard garden is preferable to a garden located adjacent to the exterior edge of the facility. If there is no other option than to install the garden on the exterior edge of the facility, eight-foot-high walls obscured by plantings will deter potential interlopers. When users can be outside with little or no supervision in a courtyard garden, unobstructed views into the garden for monitoring resident activity is necessary. In this best-case scenario, an electronic door is left open during daylight hours, so residents can come and go into the garden as they choose.

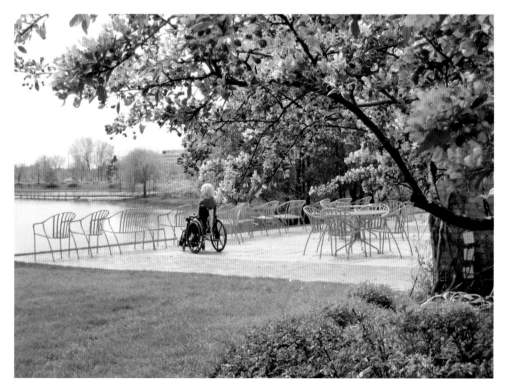

Iconic trees that shape the native environment and nourish the senses support soft fascination.

Wandering management is a vital concern. The arrangement of resident rooms around a central courtyard garden safely supports freedom of movement inside and outside. This room configuration also offers a garden view for all, including those with limited mobility. No matter where the garden is located, wayfinding cues next to its access door, such as a trellis of silk flowers or a rack with garden hats and gloves, will gently direct users to the garden.

Sensory gardens for people with dementia should be familiar and reminiscent of home. All the elements chosen, including the plants, can reconnect users to personal memories and cultural attachments. Viewing, touching, smelling, and even tasting aromatic culinary herbs may elicit long-forgotten memories and encourage social interaction and verbalization. Trees are also familiar icons, with cultural associations and attachments that will vary from region to region. Western redcedar and bigleaf maple shape the landscape of the Northwest, flowering dogwood and southern magnolia mark the South, and in tropical zones, palm trees and live oaks provide shade for sitting and resting; all convey strong regional meaning.

Walking has been shown to ease depression, a characteristic associated with dementia. For many with dementia, walking is a familiar way to engage with the world. Beyond its physiological benefits, walking stimulates exploration of natural phenomena and increases social interaction for those experiencing isolation. A single loop path with short subsidiary loops supports strolling or wheeling at a suitable pace and degree of effort. The loop can connect to an indoor circuit or simply offer an outdoor walking route. A loop with open sightlines minimizes confusion and fear of being lost.

The garden should have adequate shade and furnishings such as sturdy chairs, glider chairs (with caution), and benches with armrests strategically placed at 10- to 15-foot intervals along the loop. The clusters of seating will create natural social gathering spaces. Railings can be integrated into 36- to 38-inch-high raised beds flanking a wide, smooth, tinted concrete loop path. When raised beds abut the path, a cane tip or walker leg will not get caught off the path, the need for curbing is eliminated, and railings provide support.

Behind the raised beds install low maintenance shrubs and trees to balance the scale of the raised beds and increase near and far soft fascination benefits. The advantages of this design are multifold. It creates a natural social gathering and socializing space for small- and large-group activities and outdoor dining. It increases safety. While still rich with natural elements, users stay within the center of the garden. Every step along the route is paired with interesting plant material to view, touch, and smell. Classic herb selections that trigger pleasant memories like lavender, sage, and chamomile may be most appealing. If users choose to sit, all seating faces the flowing raised beds. Again, stable seating versus rockers and gliders may be a better option for those with dementia, as balance issues are common with older adults.

Occupational therapist Elisabeth Refn was instrumental in transforming the patio space adjacent to the front doors of UC San Diego Medical Center's Senior Behavioral Health Unit. It is now a garden she uses with patients, many of whom have dementia, other memory loss issues, and/or depression. Elisabeth repurposed the outdoor ashtrays, which happened

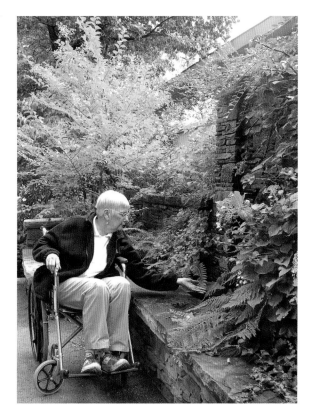

Plants to touch and smell are close at hand, and behind the raised beds, taller plantings obscure the walls of the sensory garden, providing an additional layer of visual appeal.

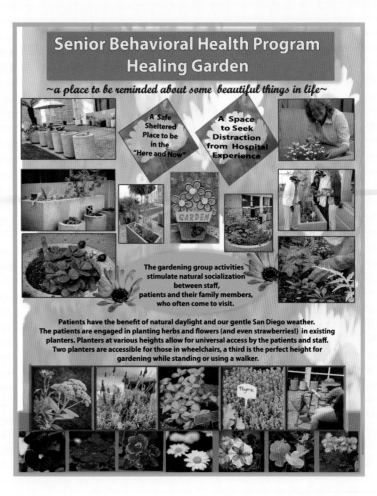

This poster for UC San Diego's therapeutic garden for seniors says and shows it all.

to be at seating height, into a series of planters filled with aromatic and tactilely rich herbs, brightly colored annuals, and tasty fruits and vegetables. She brings patients to the garden several times a week, where they can choose to tend, taste, or inhale the fragrance of the plants or to play games, socialize, or spend time in nature outside of their unit.

Imaginative elements for users to interact with may be included. For instance, an inoperable car may be appealing for those who in their younger years enjoyed tinkering. A clothesline and clothespins to peg up a basket of dish towels is a way to recreate the self-care task of hanging laundry out to dry. A carriage with a life-sized baby doll enables users to re-experience the joys of pushing a baby around the park. Tools to dig, hoe, and rake, and a broom to sweep the paths provide spontaneous opportunities to engage and do activities that may once have been important to the users. Watering cans, a push mower with the blades removed, and

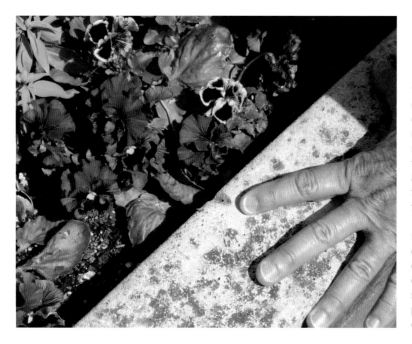

TOP For seniors and others with visual challenges, subtle notches spaced about six inches apart on the interior edge of a raised bed are a tactile spacing guide for planting.

BOTTOM Shadows cast by pergolas or overhead structures can be mistaken as steps or holes for people with dementia or low vision.

other safe (no sharp edges, not highly reflective) hand garden tools placed near raised beds may encourage users to participate in the garden. Extraneous auditory or visual stimulation, like chimes, bells, or flags are unnecessary and can be agitating. On the other hand, birdhouses hung in a backdrop trees can be sources of fascination and interest. Interaction with therapy animals is another positive sensory experience for many with dementia.

The distorted depth perception associated with age is seen most acutely in people with dementia. The shadows cast by a pergola or other overhead screening create positive and negative spaces that may look like voids or steps and become a potential tripping hazard. Some residents may avoid a pergola or overhead screen or not use the garden at all for fear of falling in the voids; thus, structures should be oriented in such a way that strong contrasts are minimized. The same response can occur with strongly contrasting paving patterns, where dark and light pavers may cause negative responses and be perceived as holes in the ground.

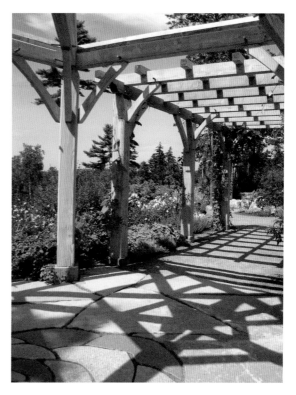

Gardens within Gardens

Sensory gardens located within botanic gardens are designed for broad appeal, not for a specific disability or condition such as ASD, PTSD, or dementia. The challenge is to design enticing sensory experiences for a wide range of visitors. A specialized sensory garden within a botanic garden may seem redundant, given that botanic gardens are intended to delight the senses. But much as they are beloved, the scope of an entire botanic garden may lead to sensory overload; and so, as with the Lerner Garden of the Five Senses at the Coastal Maine Botanical Gardens (discussed in chapter 2), the sensory garden should be sited as close to the main garden entry as possible, to attract visitors lacking the endurance, time, or patience to tour the entire garden.

The sensory garden in any context is an intimate experience. Even at a botanic garden it should not be grand or imposing but instead enticing and nourishing, an enveloping sensory experience that leaves the visitor

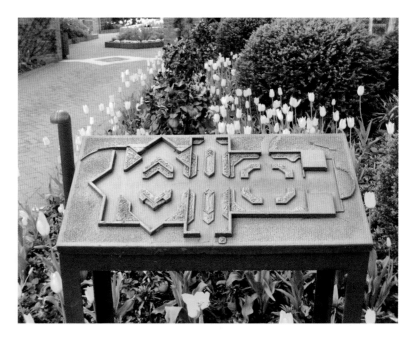

A tactile relief map is a universal design feature that orients people with visual or language challenges to the garden.

in a positive state of mind. It should also showcase universal design principles. Signage should be multisensory, to address the needs of people with sensory limitations. This includes having auditory information, a tactile relief map of the garden, and signage that combines Braille, large and clear text with a contrasting color background, and simple and consistent icons. Restrooms located in sensory gardens (or any therapeutic garden) should be clearly marked as handicapped accessible and have an electronic door opener. The garden needs to be easy to navigate, so no visitors will struggle to open a door or stretch beyond their limits to access maps, brochures, or any other garden element or material.

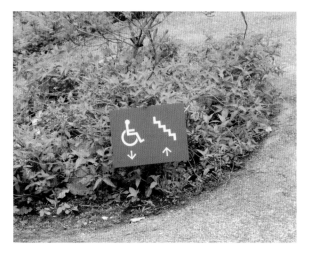

Easily understood icons direct all garden visitors and support universal design principles.

DESIGN CONSIDERATIONS

The entire site should be visually engaging in all directions and planes, with a hierarchy of views and focal points distributed throughout. Select plants in a range of colors and textures, and vary planting heights to meet the needs of all visitors, young and old, tall and short, seated or standing. For example, at the Buehler Enabling Garden at the Chicago Botanic Garden, a plethora of ever-changing flowers and herbs are strategically placed in short and tall planters, in hanging baskets accessible via pulleys, in raised beds and in vertical gardens, to be viewed and touched by sitting and standing visitors. Consider integrating sculpture or other forms of art into the design. This is a garden where anything from abstract to representational art may be appropriate because it serves a broad sector of visitors. Walls can be designed for interest through color, light and shadow, texture, and patterning, using layers of transparent screens or cutouts within a solid panel. Lighting offers dramatic and subtle visual foci and extends the benefits of the garden into the night.

The garden's overall auditory qualities need to strike a balance: too much sound can be confusing

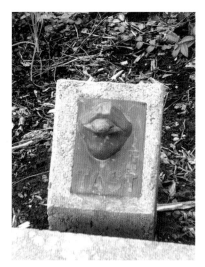

An easily recognizable sculptural icon can supplant words when demarcating a section of the sensory garden.

In addition to delineating planting spaces, walls can provide textural and visual interest in the garden.

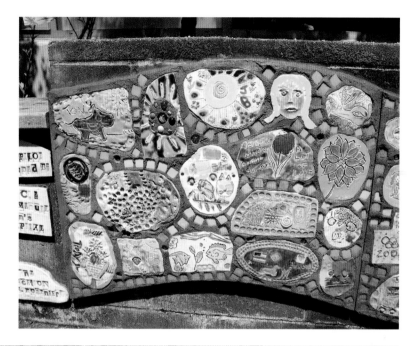

Vertically oriented musical instruments suit sitting and standing visitors equally. A clever way to ensure that the striking mallet is not lost is to build a storage caddy directly on the instrument frame.

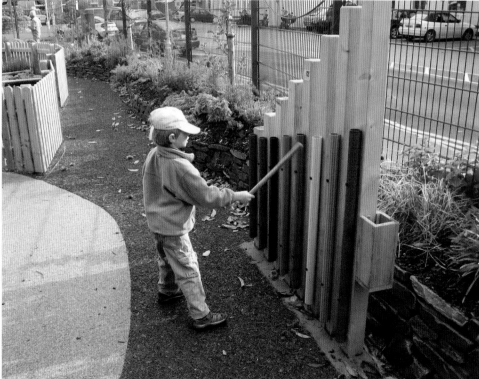

and distracting, too little may be underwhelming and uninteresting. Gentle running water offers various mesmerizing sounds and when touched provides tactile feedback. A central water feature emitting a distinctive sound can also serve as a point of orientation in the garden. Bamboo, grasses, and tree branches that shake and shimmer in the breeze emit ambient auditory experiences and can be placed throughout the garden. Bells, drums, or other instruments that can be played while seated or standing, voice conduction elements, and echo spaces all involve the garden visitor in making and receiving sounds and interacting with others. Integrated flush with a path, metallic stepping chimes that make musical sounds when feet dance, jump, or stomp on them are a great way to blend sound with movement. Such opportunities provide visitors with choices about how much and in what ways they want to engage in the sensory garden.

Olfactory experiences range from the usual subtly to strongly fragrant herbs and flowers to distinctly malodorous plant material that will delight and become a focal point for most children. The challenge is to balance scents so they do not compete with or overpower each other. Competition can lead to overstimulation and attentional fatigue. Rotating olfactory experiences with different themes (Mediterranean, culinary, medicinal) offer a variety and separation that may be more satisfying.

Taste is tricky. While a sensory garden's intention is to nourish all five basic senses, it is not practical or hygienic for visitors to snack on plants. Signage and take-home brochures that contain information about the culinary and medicinal properties of herbs may encourage visitors to plant them in their gardens, where consumption would not be an issue.

As for the sense of touch, design for surprise and variety in this garden. Smooth or rough (not too rough, though), soft or waxy—something should appeal to

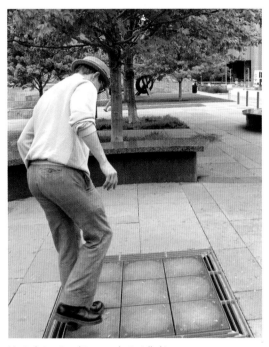

Musical stepping chimes can be installed in a sensory garden as auditory and movement elements.

Easy-to-operate or sensor-activated faucets better ensure that visitors will wash their hands before leaving the sensory garden within a garden.

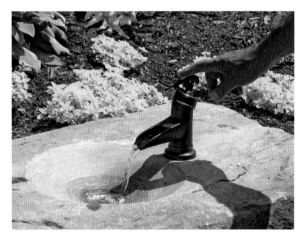

most every visitor and provide opportunities to compare and contrast the range of tactile experiences that nature provides. Water in its many expressions, still to animated, draws visitors in—to dip their fingers or wade through a shallow pool. Smooth pebbles, seeds, or pieces of sea glass can be rubbed and walked upon. If space and budget permit, install a reflexology maze or path that visitors can traverse in their bare feet or side paths with stepping stones, and tuck in a glider swing or two. Dirt for digging, ergonomic garden tools to use, and sculpture to touch are a few more tactile experiences. For the sake of practicality, site a sink with running water at the sensory garden's exit, so dirty hands can be cleaned off before visitors leave to explore the wider botanic garden.

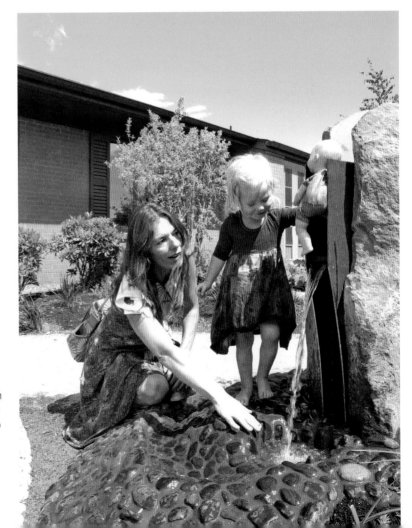

Water has broad appeal and holds great fascination for all visitors. Smooth stones glistening with water are enticing for children and adults to explore with hands and feet.

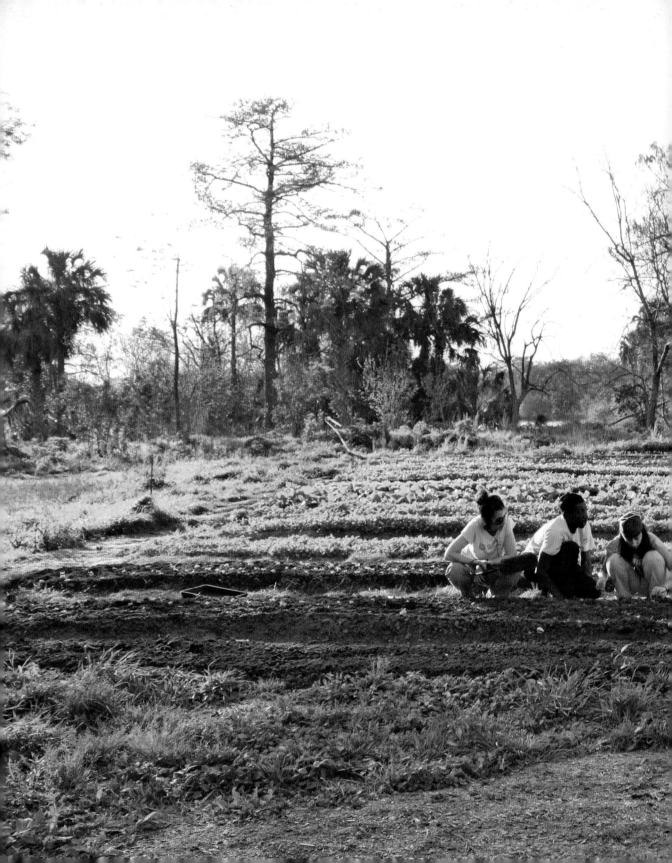

CHAPTER SEVEN

COMMUNITY GARDENS

The impulse to garden was seen in chapter 1 as a community's resilient response to the stress and isolation of wartime; later chapters explored how people dealt with war's aftermath and the continuing weights of displacement and marginalization, whatever the source, seeking solace and comfort and relearning peace in gardens. Community gardens too offer safe, supportive places to confront fears and alleviate disturbing memories. They provide both subsistence and reconnection—to other places, better times, and family life.

In the same way, although the activity remains urgent and vital for those isolated by poverty or dislocated from a familiar home landscape, communities of gardeners increasingly come together simply to build a healthier present and more sustainable future. The community gardening movement is flourishing in conjunction with rising concerns about food security and consumer concern about access to chemical-free food, but it is sometimes challenging to find the space to garden in dense urban neighborhoods, where such gardens are often most needed. Increasingly, gardeners seek non-traditional spaces to expand their operations; the rooftops of some commercial and residential buildings, car garages, restaurants, and breweries now support community gardens. Wherever they crop up—on formal sites sanctioned by municipalities and nonprofits; at houses of worship, community centers, or government agencies; on abandoned urban lots—community gardens help people find both food security and a nurturing sense of community involvement.

Shared by a Balkan war survivor: Originally I joined because of food. The garden means I don't need to go to the market and buy vegetables. It's the only income my wife and I have. I grow everything—carrot, okra, beet, tomato, cucumber, pepper, spinach, garlic, herbs, all kinds of greens, and even flowers like marigolds because the petals make good tea. Potato, onion, and cabbage are important because we live on them during winter. The garden is proof that I can still provide for us, and it gives us the feeling that we do, after all, belong somewhere. Over the years I've made friends and I find fellow chess-players here. As well as offering me food security, the garden is a place for relaxation and learning (Babbs 2011).

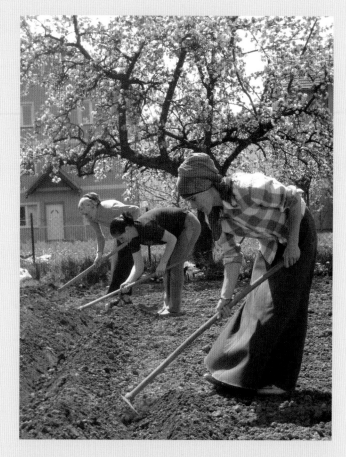

In Sarajevo, Croats, Bosniak Muslims, Serbs, and Roma now work side by side, for the common purpose of growing food to nourish their families and community.

Gardeners, artists, and activists see vacant urban lots as an opportunity for reclamation, a place to raise food and strengthen community, as here in Copenhagen.

Thriving examples of community gardens around the world showcase the many meanings of gardening in people's lives. The American Community Gardening Association, established in 1979, estimates that there are now 18,000 community gardens in the United States and Canada; internationally, the New Roots program of the International Rescue Committee advocates community gardening for refugees in 22 U.S. cities and more than 40 countries. Community gardens establish and, crucially, re-establish ties to place, culture, and food. Community gardening is all about planting a seed and growing a movement.

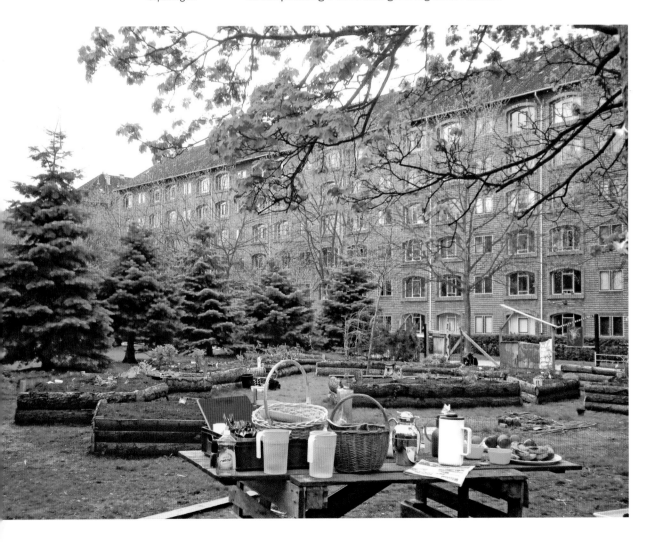

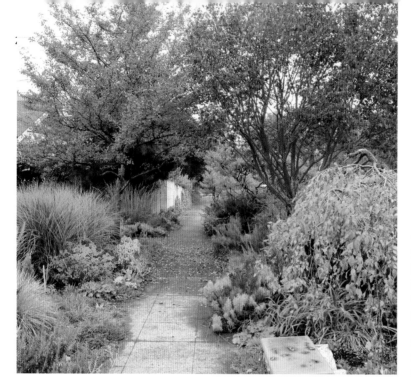

TOP Planted meridians are common in Portland, Seattle, and Vancouver, B.C. These lineal gardens increase wildlife habitat, create therapeutic green corridors in dense urban environs, and slow traffic; some are used as micro community gardens.

BOTTOM The rooftop community garden on this municipal parking garage not only has sun all day but also spectacular views.

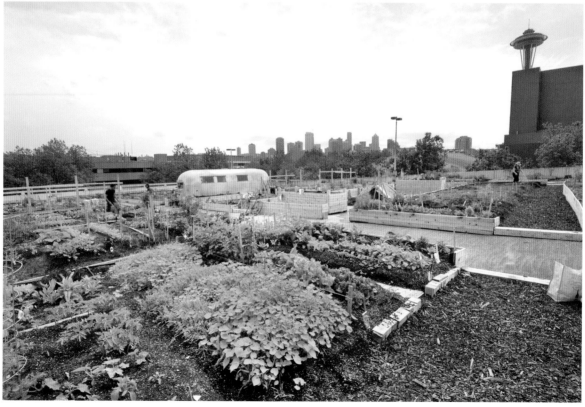

NUTRITION AND LOCAL FOOD PRODUCTION

In low-income neighborhoods where fresh vegetables and fruits are costly and hard to obtain, residents are at risk for nutrition-related illnesses such as obesity, heart disease, and diabetes. Many of these people live in apartments without access to cultivable land. The interest in breaking the cycle of disease by cultivating food is growing, as evidenced by the increasing wait periods to obtain a community garden plot.

In Florida, the nonprofit Northwood Greenlife worked with the city of West Palm Beach to create Northwood Village Greens, a small community garden on a vacant lot where rainwater from the gutters of an adjacent building is captured, diverted into two cisterns, and used to water the crops. Over in Lake Worth, the Gray Mockingbird Garden expanded from a modest community garden into a thriving CSA; Latin American vegetables are grown in a keyhole garden, and Malabar spinach climbs up over a wire-mesh tunnel that leads to raised beds and a hydroponic growing system, where lettuces and other greens are cultivated. In both places, gardeners have a designated garden to grow food while transforming unused urban spaces into a community asset—a common impetus for community gardening.

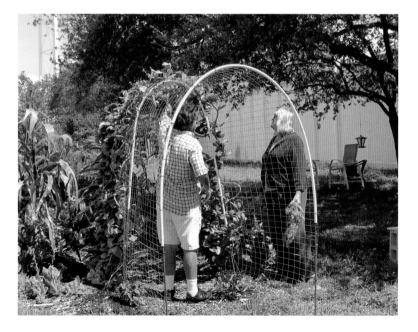

A planted archway provides support for Malabar spinach and a shady destination for gardeners in this reclaimed neighborhood gathering place.

In 2010 Seattle's P-Patch Community Gardening Program provided direct access to food for 6,300 gardeners who donated 26,248 pounds of produce to local food banks. In a 2013 P-Patch survey, 70 percent of gardeners were low income, 27 percent were people of color, 46 percent lived in apartments, and 73 percent had no gardening space where they lived. Market garden programs like P-Patch and others enable low-income and immigrant families to grow and sell their produce to the community at farm stands; gardens at senior centers provide food for older adults; and CSAs offer fresh food for urban dwellers—all are examples of how people most in need are being connected with fresh produce.

On Maui, members of the Hali'imaile Community Garden grow much of their own produce and donate to local food pantries through their Goodwill Garden. The project was a volunteer effort, building on the dream of the community outreach coordinator at Maui Land & Pineapple Company. The participants, organic gardeners all, see themselves as enriching the soil and contributing both to the health of the community and to the island's sustainability, as Hawaii imports about 90 percent of its food. The half-acre garden in the middle of sugarcane fields is surrounded by a natural eucalyptus forest. Students from the University of Hawaii Maui College cleared the spot, a former homeless encampment and dumping ground. They built a tool shed, and Maui Land & Pineapple Company provided a composting toilet, irrigation infrastructure, and a greenhouse nursery for starting seeds. Garden volunteers built and collectively tend the garden itself. A living fence features native Hawaiian trees. There is a fruit orchard and a comprehensive garden planted with culinary and medicinal herbs. In addition to the shared spaces, three primary paths, each five feet wide, provide access to the individually designated 10- by 20-foot garden plots. Repurposed eucalyptus stumps form a picnic area, and a natural gathering place is encircled with a softly rustling curtain of bamboo.

The Farmacy Garden in Fayetteville, North Carolina, offers an interesting model, integrating community gardening with healthcare and the landscaping surrounding this family medicine clinic. The hope is that the garden will improve the health and well-being of Southern Regional AHEC patients, employees, and the

A bamboo curtain creates a meditative central gathering space used for classes, resting, meals, and the occasional musical event, expanding the community garden's use and meaning.

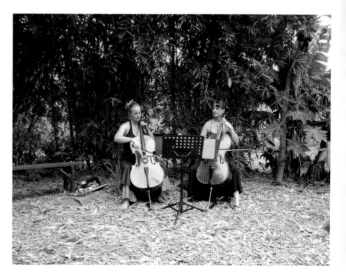

community, by increasing healthy food access through demonstration gardening and education.

Food security is a major concern on the Oregon coast, which could experience limited food access in the event of a tsunami or earthquake. Using community gardening as a strategic model for accessing healthy food in disaster scenarios is effectively demonstrated in the village of Yachats, population 700. The Yachats Community Garden, a source of inspiration and bounty, has 25 community members. The land was donated to Yachats by generous benefactors who believe in the intrinsic value of art, beauty, and sustainability. More than 10 percent of all produce grown in members' individual plots and three designated plots is donated to the local food pantry. Two beds paid for by donation are used by families who need to grow food. One bed specifically assigned to the Yachats Youth and Family Program is for preschool children to engage in sustainable gardening. Each gardener has a special attachment to the garden, and everyone participates in cleanup and keeps their garden beds camera-ready for tourists. Some members use their garden beds as a necessary source of fresh produce; some tend to their garden as a meditation, and others relish the social moments the garden can provide. Some just come to sit and ponder. Sitting in a chair that overlooks the Pacific Ocean, it is easy to feel connected to nature.

A community garden can be a place to grow, socialize, observe, and experience a sense of fulfillment.

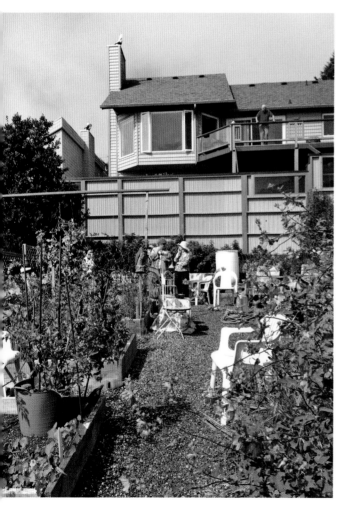

EXERCISE AND RECREATION

The activity of gardening is a purposeful exercise, and those who safely engage in it find it builds strength and restores their spirits. The physical benefits include burning calories, strengthening muscle and bone, and improving dexterity, endurance, and balance. Tilling the soil, watering, weeding, fertilizing, planting, pruning, and harvesting are complemented by the social, sensorial, and experiential pleasures of being outdoors in a verdant place.

Cantilevered beds—designed so that seated gardeners can approach the plants straight on and close to the tasks—facilitate gardening for those using wheelchairs and scooters. This design supports sound ergonomic principles, whereas standard box-shaped raised beds force seated gardeners either to position themselves sideways to garden and torque their upper bodies (which is detrimental to the musculoskeletal system) or to attempt to straddle a corner of the raised bed's edge (which limits where they can garden). Ergonomic guidelines suggest that raised beds for gardening at a kneeling position are comfortable at 12 to 18 inches in height. Accessibility heights for standing gardeners are 24 inches for children and 30 to 36 inches for adults. Optimal reach range forward is about 24 inches, so beds should not be wider than four feet. Vertical growing schemes are accessible when ergonomically designed within the limits of reach and can maximize productive yields of beans, peas, or espaliered fruit trees. Occupational therapists are well trained to understand these design principles and are an important resource to ensure a community garden is ergonomically sound.

At the Ed Benedict Community Garden in Portland, Oregon, people from Latin America, Africa, and Southeast Asia grow a cornucopia of gourds, long beans, hot peppers, exotic herbs, and potatoes. The garden, a citywide center for teaching and learning, has a series of varied-height raised beds ideal for standing located close to its entrance; while the rest of the garden has dirt paths, this portion of the garden is paved and accessible for wheelchairs or other ambulation devices.

Its center is a traditional playground, but according to Bill Dawson, Growing to Green program coordinator, the entire four-acre community garden at the Franklin Park Conservatory in Columbus, Ohio, is a playground—as well as a great example of an inclusive garden. The campus began with a collaborative design process; input was sought from neighborhood associations, block watches, local schools, governmental agencies, community gardeners, and staff. There are 40 communal gardening plots, all edged with six-inch cedar timbers to guide those with impaired vision and to keep wheeled mobility devices on the paths.

Vertical growing schemes are a good use of space and, if well designed and accessible, afford all members the gardening experience.

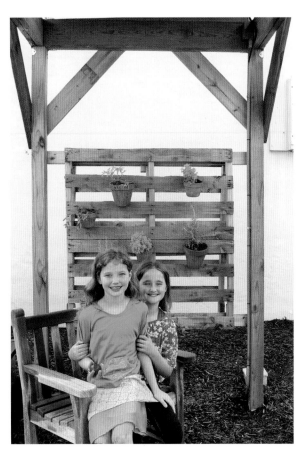

Four large raised beds are accessible by gardeners using wheelchairs or walkers, and they are proportioned for a 24-inch reach from all sides. These beds are tended by clients from Goodwill and ARC Industries, disabled veterans, and members of an intergenerational community center. Several table beds of differing heights accommodate older adults and youth. Three custom-designed tables hold removable planting containers that are used by those in wheelchairs. Various level paths—built of brick pavers, stamped concrete, decomposed granite, and stone—are all accessible.

The garden has several shade structures, many types of seating, and a serenity garden with a circular central lawn used for tai chi and other

Sustainable materials were used to create the raised beds at the Ed Benedict Community Garden.

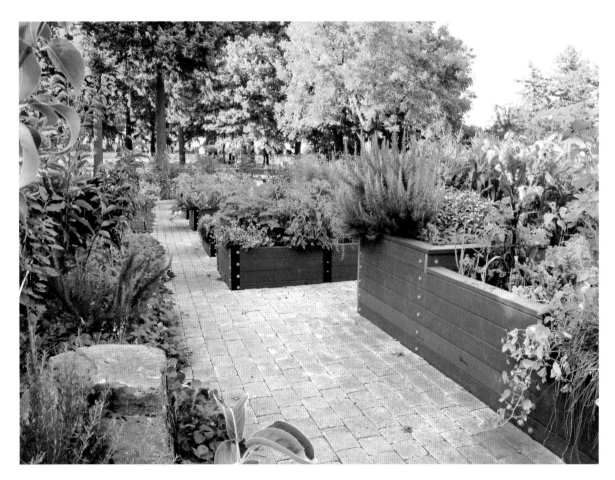

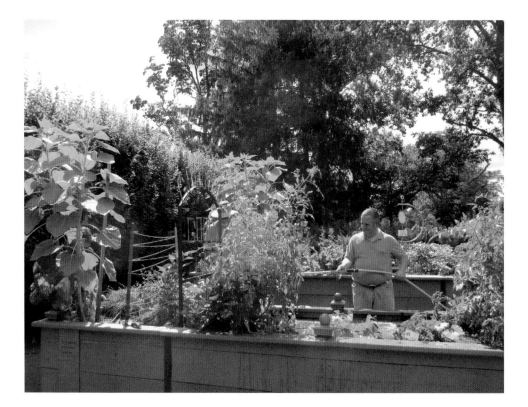

therapeutic recreation classes. Edible plants are a frequent theme; on the garden's east-west axis is a chef's allée with indoor and outdoor kitchens and a cooking theater to demonstrate wood-fired grilling and baking. Fragrance and international culinary gardens are nearby. There are fruit trees and a berry yard and house with screen walls to admit pollinators and deter birds. Compost bins, an apiary, and pollinator's plantings enhance the fertility of these gardens, which provide 3,000 pounds of food a year to a local soup kitchen. The campus has a gardener training program, and this artfully designed and energetic place is appropriately the national headquarters for the American Community Gardening Association.

Tending raised beds is just one part of the Growing to Green program at Franklin Park Conservatory and Botanical Gardens.

NATURAL CYCLES AND PERMACULTURE

Community gardens beautify neighborhoods and create a world apart from the civic concerns and everyday occupations of the built environment. The garden in turn tunes people to the natural cycles as they enter, preserve, and care for green space. Through seasonal changes and vagaries of weather, a sequence of hands-on tasks unfolds and, at times, surges all at once. Community gardeners share and celebrate these moments,

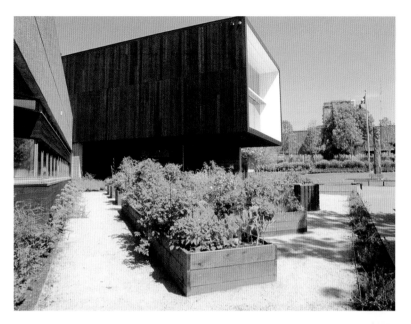

RIGHT Community gardens at municipal buildings soften the institutional sense and link nature with the built environment. This one marks the entry to North Vancouver City Hall.

BELOW People gather, recreate, and garden in this vibrant civic space outside Vancouver City Hall through all the seasons of the year.

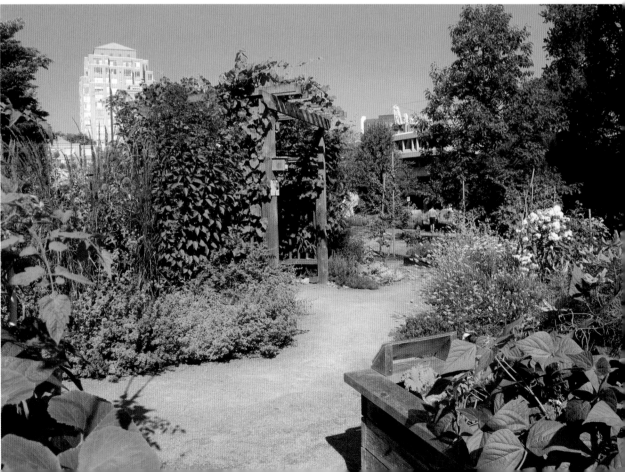

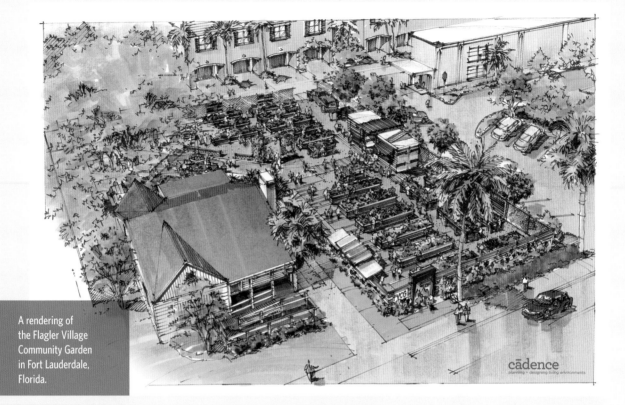

A rendering of the Flagler Village Community Garden in Fort Lauderdale, Florida.

planting seeds or starts, pruning grapes and fruit trees, picking berries, and harvesting vegetables. Many growing communities further connect gardeners from harvest to food preservation, cooking, and healthy eating.

A garden board in Fort Lauderdale reclaimed a plot of land in an effort to preserve the city's natural beauty and inspire its cultural revitalization. The resulting Flagler Village Community Garden, founded on the principles of growing, reflecting, exploring, and engaging within the community, is designed with longevity and usability in mind. Circulation paths, raised beds, secure equipment storage, spaces for demonstrations, and a shaded common area all make for a comfortable atmosphere for socializing as well as gardening. Cadence served as garden master planner and landscape architect of record for the project.

Organic gardeners balance their cultivating strategies and interventions with letting nature take its course. This is a mindful way of gardening that invites participants to pay attention, closely observe, and learn from experience. Gardeners attend to the fertility or tilth of the soil and the cycling of nutrients through vermiculture and composting. They respect beneficial insects and pollinators. They select and rotate a diversity of plants well adapted to their growing conditions, and reject the use of toxic pesticides and herbicides used in industrial agriculture.

Permaculture, another holistic approach to cultivating food, emerged as a reaction to industrial agriculture and its legacy: reduced biodiversity, increased loss of topsoil, and a dependence on nonrenewable resources and chemical fertilizers. Proponents view permaculture as an ecologically responsible form of agriculture that focuses on the interrelationships between its various components to achieve a high level of synergy. Keyhole gardens, for example, make use of permaculture principles, as the bed is filled with layers of dirt and compostable materials; the central composting bin helps keep the soil moist, while the structure itself helps to regulate the temperature of the soil and prevent erosion that would be inevitable in an at-grade garden bed.

Ruth McLean, an Australian landscape architect now living in New Zealand, feels that permaculture can be applied to any outdoor space, from a balcony to a cityscape or community garden. A site she designed

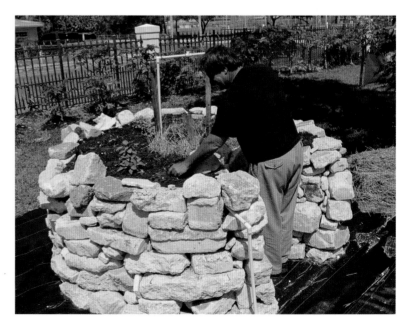

Keyhole gardens link social and environmental sustainability. Completely customizable, they are an efficient way to integrate composting and growing.

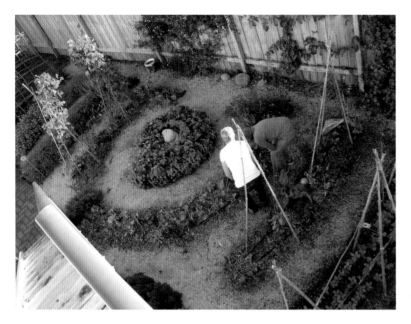

Although sometimes associated with being unruly and untidy, with careful planning a permaculture garden can be a work of beauty.

for client Marie Manning, an avid gardener originally from Canada, is small by New Zealand standards, approximately 320 square feet of a suburban backyard. The design brief included a desire to provide sustenance for body, mind, and spirit (it is a big thrill for Marie, in her new climate, to be able to harvest food from the garden every day of the year). The garden's rippling circular pattern offers a "centering" gesture and recalls the Uretara River, which flows nearby; the small stone assemblage in its center references the Inukshuk constructions of Canada's Inuit people.

The vegetable bed system borrows heavily from John Jeavons's work on biointensive cropping as well as from leading New Zealand organic gardener Kay Baxter. Note that the garden plan uses the word "permablitz," an Australian term for a permacultural makeover that builds community resilience through sharing information, sharing labor, sharing food, and sharing fun. This social agenda is at the heart of many permaculture projects, which can be summed up in three ethical principles: earthcare, people care, and fair share. In practice, it meant that the transformation of this yard from lawn to food production took place on one Saturday with the help of about 20 volunteers. The model is that if you attend three permablitzes, you are entitled to host one at your place.

A natural, functional, mature ecosystem thrives due to the interdependency of its many layers. Just so, permaculture is focused on multiple layers: canopy, understory, shrubs, herbaceous, soil surface (including cover crops, green manures, and organic matter), rhizosphere, and a vertical

OPPOSITE A plan for a permaculture garden in New Zealand.

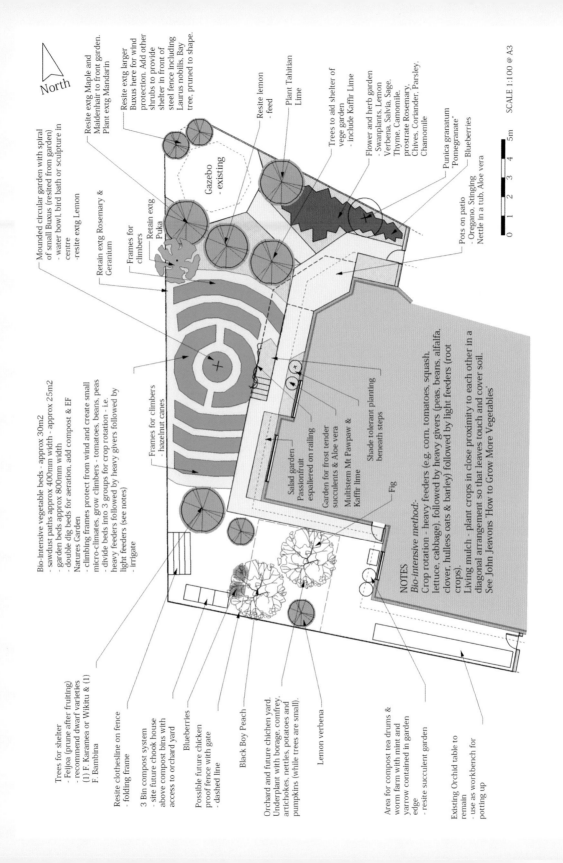

North

SCALE 1:100 @ A3

0 1 2 3 4 5m

Mounded circular garden with spiral of small Buxus (resited from garden)
- water bowl, bird bath or sculpture in centre
- resite extg Lemon

Resite extg larger Buxus here for wind protection. Add other shrubs to provide shelter in front of steel fence including Laurus nobilis. Bay tree, pruned to shape.

Resite extg Maple and Maidenhair to front garden. Plant extg Mandarin

Resite lemon - feed

Plant Tahitian Lime

Trees to aid shelter of vege garden - include Kaffir Lime

Flower and herb garden - Swanplants. Lemon Verbena. Salvia. Sage. Thyme. Camomile. prostrate Rosemary, Chives. Coriander, Parsley. Chamomile

Punica granatum "Pomegranate"

Blueberries

Pots on patio - Oregano. Stinging Nettle in a tub. Aloe vera

Retain extg Rosemary & Geranium

Frames for climbers

Retain extg Puka

Gazebo - existing

Bio-Intensive vegetable beds - approx 30m2
- sawdust paths approx 400mm width - approx 25m2
- garden beds approx 800mm width
- double dig beds for aeration. add compost & EF Natures Garden
- climbing frames protect from wind and create small micro-climates, grow climbers - tomatoes, beans, peas
- divide beds into 3 groups for crop rotation - i.e. heavy feeders followed by light givers followed by light feeders (see notes)
- irrigate

Frames for climbers - hazelnut canes

Salad garden Passionfruit espaliered on railing

Garden for frost tender succulents & Aloe vera

Multistem Mt Pawpaw & Kaffir lime

Shade tolerant planting beneath steps

Fig

NOTES
Bio-intensive method:-
Crop rotation - heavy feeders (e.g. corn, tomatoes, squash, lettuce, cabbage). followed by heavy givers (peas, beans, alfalfa, clover, hulless oats & barley) followed by light feeders (root crops).
Living mulch - plant crops in close proximity to each other in a diagonal arrangement so that leaves touch and cover soil.
See John Jeavons 'How to Grow More Vegetables'

Trees for shelter
- Feijoa (prune after fruiting)
- recommend dwarf varieties (1) F. Karamea or Wikitu & (1) F. Bambina

Resite clothesline on fence
- folding frame

3 Bin compost system
- site future chook house above compost bins with access to orchard yard

Blueberries

Possible future chicken proof fence with gate
- dashed line

Black Boy Peach

Orchard and future chichen yard. Underplant with borage. comfrey. artichokes, nettles, potatoes and pumpkins (while trees are small).

Lemon verbena

Area for compost tea drums & worm farm with mint and yarrow contained in garden edge
- resite succulent garden

Existing Orchid table to remain
- use as workbench for potting up

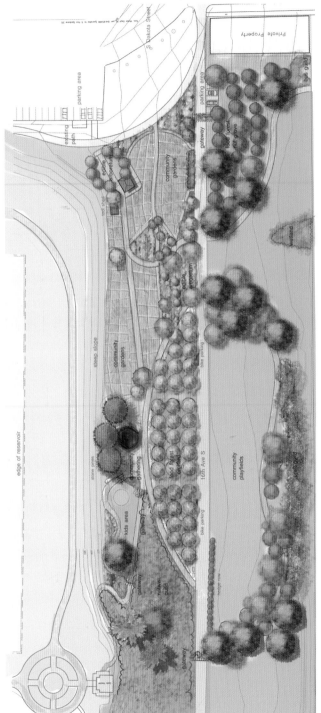

A schematic site plan of Seattle's Beacon Food Forest.

layer made up of vines. Some proponents include an eighth layer, fungi, to complete the three-dimensional "food forest."

Permaculture offers multiple benefits to the overall health and welfare of the planet. Permaculture does not offer all the benefits desired from a therapeutic garden or the goals of universal access, physical rehabilitation, and therapeutic horticulture. What permaculture does provide is a foundational principle upon which other goals related to garden design can be integrated without harming the earth or creating waste.

A recent example of merging the principles of permaculture and community gardening is found in the seven-acre Beacon Food Forest, a new model of community gardening based on the principles of permaculture, urban farming, and land stewardship. The design and development process was inclusive and participatory. Several workshops attended by local residents, permaculturalists, community gardeners, and ecological advocacy groups were held to solicit ideas and review the designs; translators assisted residents of the diverse Seattle neighborhood of Beacon Hill, many of whom speak no English. The design strives to improve the health of the community by integrating ethical harvesting, education, recreation, and habitat creation into the food forest. It features edible arboretums with fruits from around the globe, a food forest orchard, a food forest nut grove, and community playfields, as well as traditional allotment plots. The whole results in reclamation of native habitat as a multilayer, edible forest garden. The reestablishment of trees on the site will, in a modest way, also reduce climate impacts by providing shade and reducing carbon dioxide.

LEARNING AND SKILL DEVELOPMENT

As described in chapter 5, a garden can be a transformative learning environment. Community gardens are increasingly being used by afterschool programs. For youth lacking positive, stable role models, the garden is a place where older peers or adults become mentors. Students learn not just gardening but also leadership skills; they mediate conflicts and organize productive work parties. Through the meaningful task of growing healthy food for their neighbors, young people are inspired to become activists for personal, social, and environmental change in their communities.

At Grow Dat Youth Farm, a diverse group of high school students recruited from local schools complete a 20-week job training program

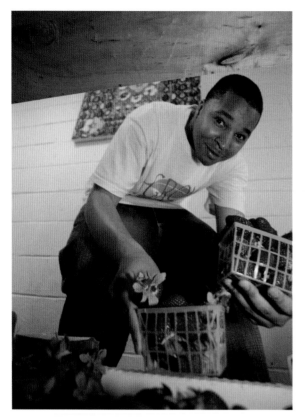

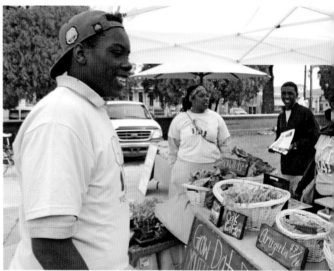

LEFT It is a sweet deal: growing, harvesting, and preparing ripe red strawberries for sale or distribution to local homeless and underserved populations.

BELOW Students at Grow Dat Youth Farm are proud to talk about the fruits of their labor at local farmers' markets.

that focuses on building excellence in leadership, agriculture, wellness, and food justice—learned skills that are intended to lead to future employment in the urban agriculture sector. Grow Dat is situated on four acres of a New Orleans public park, along a bayou defined by native cypress and live oaks. The campus includes indoor and outdoor classrooms, offices, wash and storage facilities, and a two-acre organic farm. The site, a former golf course, was developed by Tulane City Center, an outreach program of Tulane University's School of Architecture, using recycled shipping containers. The bright green containers were elevated to avoid flooding and modified for energy efficiency; they are stacked and linked by skyways and decking.

Seattle Youth Garden Works, a program of Seattle Tilth, is an after-school job training and education program for youth who are homeless or at risk of dropping

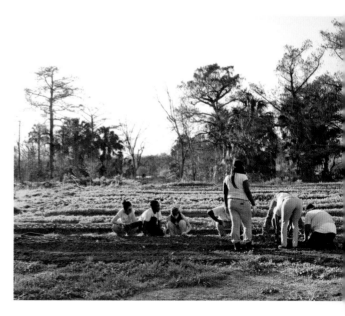

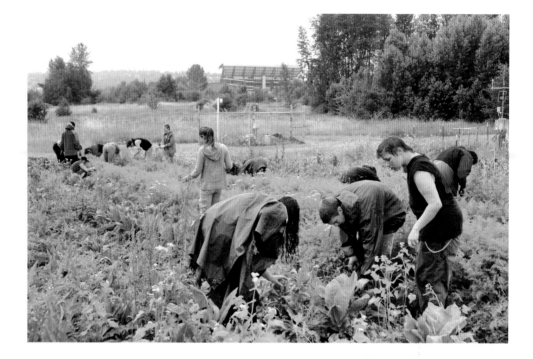

At the Seattle Youth Garden Farm, youth walk up and down the rows with clippers, knives, and baskets, harvesting zucchini, squash, and pole beans.

OPPOSITE, BOTTOM Work teams come together to prepare a planting bed at the Grow Dat Youth Farm. Working collaboratively fosters trust, interdependence, and increases self-confidence.

out of school, and the community farm is their outdoor classroom. Participants are paid a modest stipend to plant, grow, harvest, and sell their produce at local farmers' markets, all the while acquiring meaningful experience in urban agriculture. For many, it is their first exposure to nature and gardening, not to mention personal responsibility and teamwork. Participants spend half their time working at the farm and green market stand and the other half in classes focusing on nutrition and business and leadership skills. The farm is adjacent to the University of Washington's Center for Urban Horticulture; it is a nonthreatening, green sanctuary where gang violence and the temptation to engage in deviant behavior are absent. Enthusiasm for gardening may be perceived as being "uncool" in their home environments, but when at the farm the youth embrace it, and their shared endeavor unites them. Deep and unique bonds of trust form between group members, strengthening self-identity and building confidence and sense of mastery. Staff and mentors not only instruct the youth but serve as role models, providing guidance, connecting them to housing and social services, and troubleshooting problems to ensure they stay in school. The mentoring and support the youth receive may be the critical component that transforms their lives for the better.

In South Carolina, Lowcountry Local First's Growing New Farmers program trains the next generation of farmers in three phases:

apprenticeships, farm incubation, and links to afford-able land. Dirt Works, the first incubator farm, is currently home to seven new farmers. Participants lease an acre of land for $2,000 a year and have access to a tractor, packing shed, walk-in cooler, tool storage, irrigation, and a mentor farmer to apprentice with. Farmers have three years in the program to refine their plan, build their market, and save capital to launch their businesses. An additional acre of Dirt Works is reserved as a teaching plot, where the public can learn core farming concepts and innovative techniques. The teaching acre includes raised beds, the purpose of which is twofold: the project itself is inclusive, and community members can see examples of how to make their home gardens inclusive.

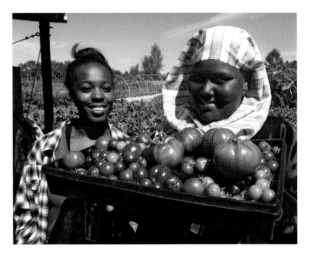

Growing, harvesting, and sharing produce with the wider community transforms the lives of Seattle Youth Garden Works participants.

FRIENDSHIP AND BELONGING

Another therapeutic outcome cultivated in community gardens is the positive psychological benefit gained through participation, work, ritual, and celebration. For those experiencing marginalization, low self-esteem, and a sense of inefficacy, an improved sense of self-worth is elicited through the shared endeavors of planting, growing, harvesting, cooking, and eating. Many community gardens are structured around individual plots, where the sense of accomplishment and empowerment are aligned with individual development. This model yields a vast tapestry of different types of food, often reflective of the ethnic and cultural backgrounds of the growers. In the communal model, responsibility falls to participants to work together, and through the process of resolving conflict and discussing acceptable behavior and responsibilities, a deeper level of community is created.

Through participation in a community garden, emotional connections or attachments are formed, a sense of belonging cultivated, and identification to one's culture reinforced. This is especially important for immigrants and refugees, many of whom have experienced severe and traumatic displacement from their homelands. Recreating or adapting a place to reestablish a sense of familiarity can ease the transition from the familiar to unfamiliar, thus reducing stresses resulting from these difficult transitions.

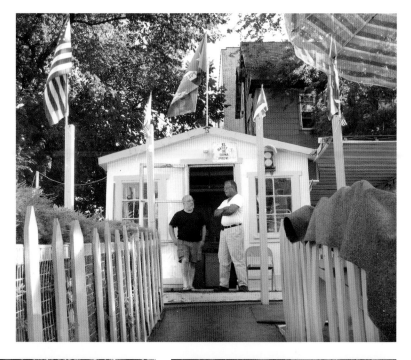

The open space at El Batey de Dona Provi Community Garden is used for ad hoc recreations, rituals, celebrations, and gatherings. For many Puerto Ricans in the Bronx, this casita is the community center of choice.

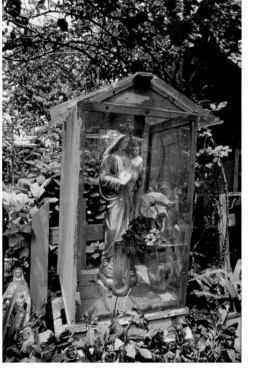

LEFT The iconography and images painted on a variety of surfaces, when combined with masks and folk art, complete the transformation of place into a space of belonging.

RIGHT For others in the community, the visual intrigue, tropical abundance of vegetation, and reclamation of space inspires curiosity, spurring cross-cultural exchange of information, food, and stories.

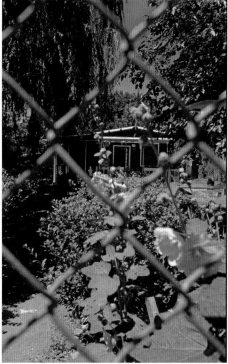

The casita of urban Puerto Rican neighborhoods differs significantly from "traditional" community gardens in its use and purpose. While the primary activity of most community gardens is cultivation of produce and ornamental plantings, the casita also serves as classroom, daycare/play area, performance space, ceremonial space, and community center. Casitas are created by a user group united by common cultural heritage, and through the gardens their community identity is reinforced. The gardens are an aesthetic, social, and spiritual oasis and reflection of their community. They consist of edible, ornamental, and medicinal plantings along with opportunistic species, presenting a contrast of wild and cultivated—the whole offering a natural counterpoint to the hardness of the environment and an essential place to relax. Both being within the garden and the act of cultivating it are effective for reducing anxiety.

As a place, every aspect of the casita expresses Puerto Rican culture, whether that expression is in the form of indigenous architecture, visual arts, music, dance, or social life. These elements, woven together, form the experiential and metaphorical sense of place—all are components of a cultural landscape, a "home." They are also evocative for those on the "other side" of the fence: many passersby, unaware of the Puerto Rican culture, are drawn to the strong, vibrant naturalness of casitas, which transcends cultural barriers and taps more universal meanings. Murals painted by members complete the casita's transformation. Rest in peace murals, akin to the actual burials that consecrate homeowner's yards in rural Puerto Rico, are a common feature, as are images of hometown scenes and renderings of the coqui, the island's iconic tree frog.

In neighborhoods where safety is a concern, an accessible community garden can become a desirable place to come together with the common goal of growing and feeding the local community.

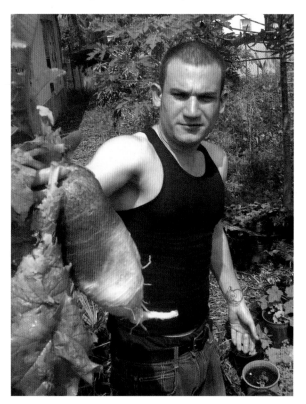

CRIME AND ISSUES OF SAFETY

In distressed neighborhoods with prevailing unemployment and high rates of crime, community gardens offer safe havens of order, civility, and productive work. As one plot is cultivated, it has a ripple effect; other plots are revitalized, leading to a network of enhanced green spaces and more active social engagement and

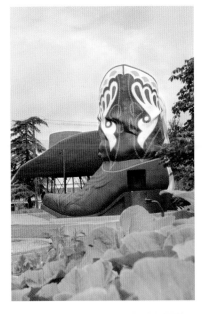

community resiliency. Crime rates are reduced in neighborhoods with a community garden. Community gardens are neutral territories, where nature harbors few threats and where those experiencing loss, disconnection, and trauma find refuge from their fears and stressors.

FUNDING

Landscape designers often design community gardens as pro-bono projects, but grant funding sources are available to those looking for compensation. Check with the American Community Gardening Association, as well as city, county, and state governments and the more than 1,400 community foundations, which among other services have searchable funding databases. A simple online search pairing "community foundation" with the proposed garden's town (or closest large municipality) should lead to a local community foundation.

ABOVE When budgets are tight, make use of salvaged and recycled material. In Oxbow Park, another P-Patch community garden, a hat and boots (formerly a gas station and restroom, respectively) now serve as a gathering pavilion and upgraded restroom and storage shed.

RIGHT Many people find meaning and purpose in building a community garden from the ground up, gratis. The sense of ownership and pride is there from the start.

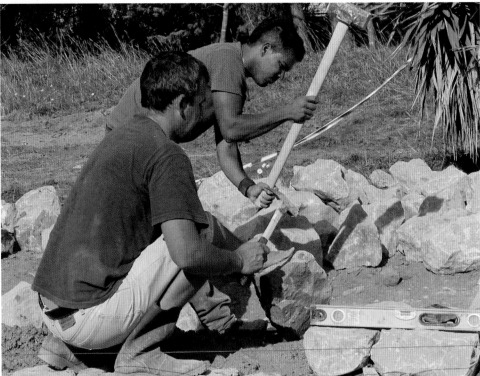

DESIGN CONSIDERATIONS

Involving an interdisciplinary design team in the community design process focuses participants on inclusiveness and accountability and on the best practices of design and safe gardening. When designing a community garden, all applicable municipal regulations should be understood and followed and required permits obtained prior to construction. Many regulations pertain to ADA access, health and safety issues, and guidelines for heights and setbacks of structures. Working with community organizers to create hands-on educationally focused community gardens that meet the needs of the homeless and impoverished is a niche practice area for interdisciplinary design teams.

An environment that supports learning and social engagement requires spaces that are comfortable, ecological, and engaging. Participants need protection from the elements, spaces to accommodate the largest groups, and areas for smaller gatherings and intimate social exchanges. Seating serves dual purposes; it must be sturdy yet movable, allowing gardeners

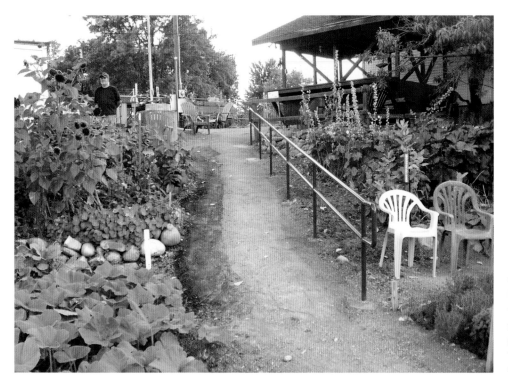

Movable and flexible seating and handrails increase the inclusivity and safety of a community garden and are more welcoming to people of varying abilities.

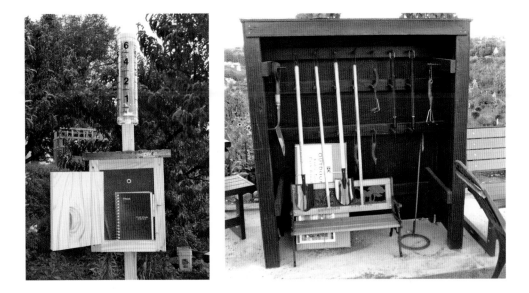

LEFT The welfare and viability of a community garden is increased when important information is made readily available to its growers.

RIGHT A well-organized tool shed makes it easy to keep track of tools and sends a positive message of pride in maintaining the beauty of the garden. This one is also a small place to wait out a summer shower.

to choose where they sit and to rearrange the space to meet their needs. Space, user needs, and budget impact what is included in a community garden; common elements are tool sheds with wheelchair access, composting and material storage areas, multiple water faucets, vegetable cleaning tables, announcement boards or kiosks, and covered gathering spaces.

Many community gardens are enhanced with functional and decorative art, vehicles for personal and cultural expression. Often this is vernacular art made from salvaged materials; such art is temporal, original, and cathartic for the gardeners. ADA paths should accommodate both wheeled mobility devices and wheelbarrows with a minimum width of five feet. A more generous path eight feet in width could allow a pickup truck filled with compost or mulch to make a delivery to the garden. Urban sites, though often relatively small, can through creative design have expansive gardening opportunities; vertical-trellised walls provide structures for climbing vines, arbors support grapes and kiwi, and green wall systems with stacked planter boxes or grow bags are ideal for tomatoes, herbs, and other vegetables. All facilitate maximum production in limited spaces.

Plants should be selected for their IPM (integrated pest management) benefits. Plants hosting beneficial insects are incorporated into the garden to control problematic insects that damage the crops. Native plants

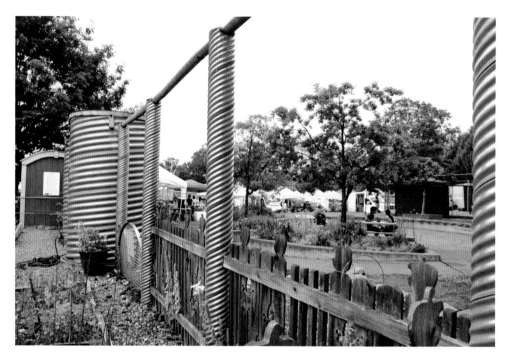

Fencing can be both attractive and creative while defining the community garden's perimeter. It can also be used to support trellising fruits and vegetables and integrated as a rainwater conveyance system.

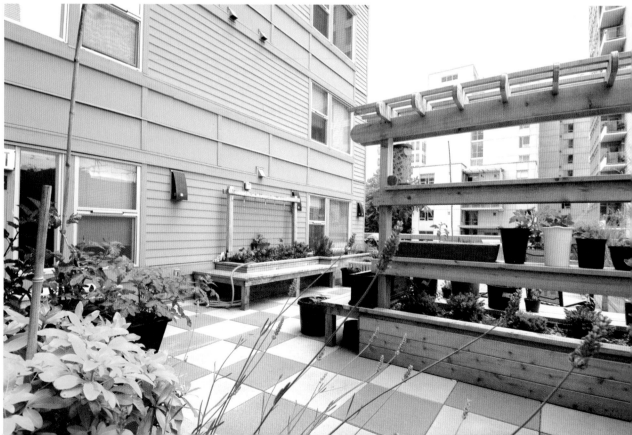

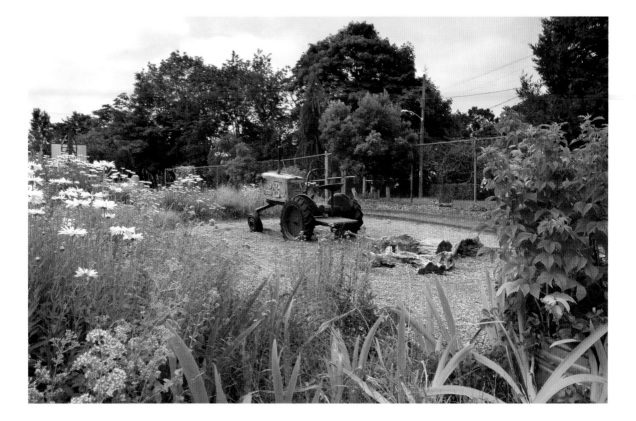

Creativity is the norm when designing appealing playscapes for children at community gardens. They are usually an assortment of natural and found objects, only seldom a manufactured structure.

OPPOSITE A series of raised beds with vertical trellising increases the type and variety of plants that can be grown and harvested at this transitional housing courtyard.

increase habitat value, attracting birds and other species, and offering learning opportunities and interest for users of all ages. In some community gardens meeting spaces for classes and modest play areas are incorporated to increase community gathering and support children's activities while adult family members tend their plots. Playscapes are often unconventional (old farm machinery, building materials) or made from natural materials (logs, stepping stumps, rocks); trees are for climbing and a thicket of shrubs makes for creative exploration.

CLOSER LOOK

IHCC–MSU Interdisciplinary Community Garden and Orchard

Student gardeners from two Minnesota schools, Inver Hills Community College and Metropolitan State University, did it all when it came to their community garden. They designed and built the garden shed; they routed signs, grouted tiles and bricks, and stained all the wood. The garden consists of three areas. In the first two, an apple orchard and a community garden, students and faculty work together to grow produce destined for local shelters and food pantries; the third area is a traditional garden of individual allotments where, typically, neighbors grow food for themselves and their families in 10- by 10-foot plots and share abundant harvests with the larger community. Everything is grown without pesticides, and an outdoor classroom adjacent to the garden is wheelchair-accessible. The plan is to have local Boy Scouts build raised plots so those with physical challenges will not have to bend over while gardening.

Students work and volunteer for a variety of reasons, the main one being that they enjoy doing something positive for the community while also learning in the process. The garden provides stress relief for them—it makes them feel good to get out of the classroom and to work outdoors, with and for others. Growing food for underserved people is a central theme of a course August Hoffman, professor of psychology at MSU, teaches in community psychology, and several of his students volunteer to help such individuals.

In 2013, the garden partnered with LifeWorks, a nonprofit serving people with disabilities. Adult

One of the student-driven projects was working with adults with developmental disabilities to build a tool shed.

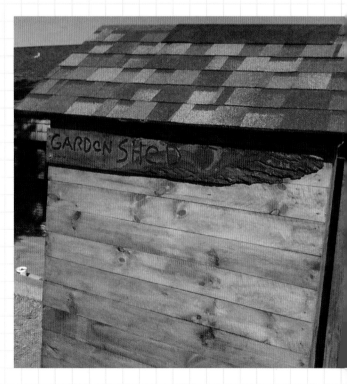

At this community garden, college students work with community members to build infrastructure and grow and share produce with local food pantries.

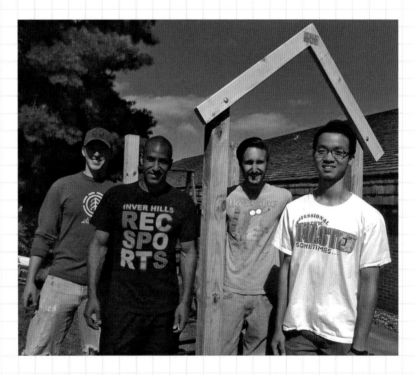

clients came out every Wednesday during the growing season to help with watering. These new gardeners are as committed as the students are to giving back to the community, according to Barbara Curchack, professor of psychology at IHCC and, with August, co-coordinator of the community garden and orchard. That year, the garden donated 1,169 pounds of fresh fruit and vegetables to two food shelves, Eagan-Lakeville Resource Center and Neighbors, Inc., as well as to St. Paul Lutheran Church.

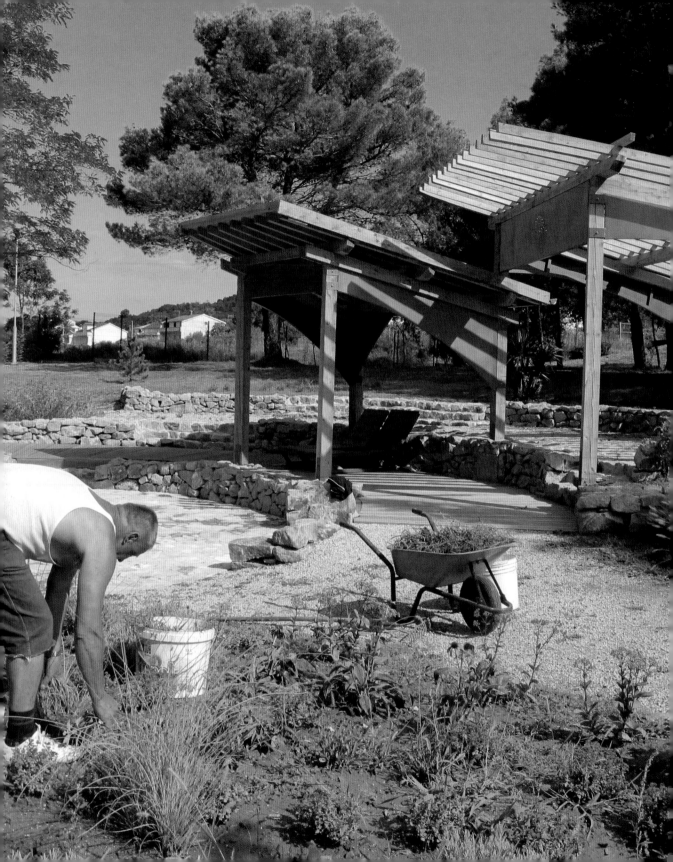

CHAPTER EIGHT

MAINTAINING THE THERAPEUTIC GARDEN

Feasible maintenance, both of plants and of hardscape, is the key to a well-designed therapeutic garden being used to its maximal potential. It is essential to consider this aspect at the beginning of planning and design. A healthy, thriving landscape and the healing benefits expected for its users fundamentally derive from ongoing care and stewardship. How this will be managed and by whom, with how much time and expertise and at what cost, will guide the scope of the project and help it to unfold in successful stages.

At a psychiatric hospital in Rab, Croatia, patients now maintain the garden they helped to design and install, as part of an occupational therapy program. The work itself is therapeutic, providing a distraction from problems and even improved sleep patterns.

Planning for Maintenance

A first priority to establish with prospective clients is to determine who will be maintaining the garden. The garden may be cared for by onsite facilities maintenance, contracted out, or in part maintained by therapists, patients, and volunteers. Each of these scenarios presents a different picture for the garden's cultivation and maintenance. Knowing the options available will enable a designer to match the needs of the garden with the available resources of the facility. One thing is certain: having a variety of participants care for the garden has many benefits for those receiving formal therapy and for those who are working in the garden for the sheer pleasure of being outdoors. Working together for the common purpose of maintaining it builds a sense of community around the therapeutic garden.

Gathering facility personnel, resident, and volunteer input during the design process is invaluable and establishes a sense of shared team effort that returns social, economic, and ecological dividends once the project has been completed and maintenance is ready to be addressed. A sizable therapeutic garden will generate a community of supporters to pool and coordinate expertise, effort, and learning to maintain it. The community may include therapists, patients, volunteers, and maintenance staff, in-house or contracted seasonally. Some facilities will have the resources to hire a maintenance company to oversee the long-term care of the garden. If so, it will be important to involve them in the design process; they bring extensive experience to the design team, and that experience can help you avoid problems they have encountered in previous jobs.

If staff personnel (including facilities management and therapy staff) would like to take on additional tasks, it is important to establish whether they have the work force, budget, time, and knowledge to take on this responsibility. A therapist's specific role in the horticultural aspect of garden maintenance is to train and supervise interested patients to undertake tasks that align with their therapy goals and are within their safe scope of abilities. Therapists may also train and supervise volunteers, who, unlike patients, are not working within the scope of a therapy program. If the garden is installed at a long-term care facility, residents who are not receiving formal therapy may also want to be involved with maintenance; their voice, too, is important in the participatory design process: determine their level of interest and skill (and, if necessary, establish how they will be provided with the proper training if skills are lacking).

Sometimes maintenance will be entirely dependent on volunteer groups such as master gardeners, local schools, garden clubs, or retirees. These contributors can be very effective and many bring deep knowledge, but recognize that such groups often have a high rate of turnover, and many volunteers are unavailable in the summer. Volunteers may also work under the supervision of facilities maintenance staff. In either case, even the most seasoned volunteers will benefit from training to do horticultural chores using sound ergonomic techniques; workshops led by occupational or physical therapists will make certain that eager volunteers at all skill levels understand proper lifting and movement techniques and avoid physical injury.

Appropriate design choices and the human capital needed to maintain the garden directly influence whether the garden will be used to meet therapeutic objectives or fall into disuse because it is impossible to care for. Those responsible for overseeing the garden's maintenance must understand the objectives and maintenance requirements of the garden, so their efforts or supervision of contracted workers will ensure that hardscape elements are kept in safe working order. At the same time, there can and should be a division of labor. Accessible planting beds mean that the garden will in part be maintained by patients and staff. Try to avoid high-maintenance horticultural choices like topiaries, clipped hedges, and unruly plants. Select plantings that will benefit from a significantly lower level of attention, needing perhaps only deadheading, light pruning, and routine propagating and replanting. Many annuals and herbaceous perennials are good options to include in a therapeutic garden that patients, therapists, and volunteers will take ownership of (in turn, reducing the burden on facilities maintenance).

The design team can present ideas to clients with a clear outline of the associated budgets of time and money needed to keep the garden serviceable and healthy. Understanding the implications of the design and material choices comes from practical experience that facility owners and managers may not possess. Engaging with facility personnel (for example, including them in design review meetings) can build their understanding and investment, leading to a appropriate design with a plan for care and stewardship in place for the long term. The challenge for designers is to create design proposals that a client can realistically maintain and fund.

The completed project will require supervision to oversee a schedule of assigned responsibilities in two areas, plant maintenance and hardscape maintenance. Depending on location and season, some maintenance tasks will need attention daily or several times weekly. Safety checks—such as making sure that paths are kept free of tripping hazards like fallen branches and hoses, or looking to see that water features are not over-flowing or leaking—need to be done daily. Other frequent maintenance tasks may include watering, mowing, light pruning, staking, deadhead-ing, and harvesting. Seasonal maintenance tasks include fertilizing, heavy pruning, and inspection of structures, paving, and irrigation, drainage, and lighting systems.

Finally, a designer should provide clients with a two-part (plant and hardscape) maintenance manual for their particular therapeutic garden. The first part typically outlines the care of planting areas, with general information on feeding, weeding, watering, and pruning; a garden calen-dar, breaking down the tasks seasonally, and a plant list organized by type (groundcovers, perennials, shrubs, trees) are also included. It's a good idea to cite further resources for plant maintenance—regional guides to plants and handbooks to address pest and disease problems, for exam-ple. The section on hardscape maintenance and repair will address sys-tems (such as for irrigation) that have specific operating instructions and components that might need replacement; the section on lighting, for example, will list bulbs by the manufacturer's item number. For all sys-tems, operating diagrams will show settings for timers and sensors, and locations of shutoffs and drains or valves. The manual should also list any system installers and material vendors and suppliers.

Plant Maintenance

Plant maintenance in a therapeutic garden is much like the care of any other kind of garden. If plants are selected using regional guides and suggested lists from county extension programs, master gardener associations, and water utilities, they will be appropriate for temperature, zone, drought, and soil types, and the garden will be maintained with less effort. Cautionary lists of invasive plants should be consulted, as nurseries sometimes euphemistically label such plants as "vigorous." Vines and groundcovers in particular can be rampant, requiring frequent pruning or containment of underground roots systems. Perennials like lemon balm (*Melissa officinalis*) and oregano (*Origanum vulgare*) can self-sow widely, becoming hard to control. Probably the most notorious land-grabber is any running bamboo. Recommended lists will offer the therapeutic garden a trove of hardy, adaptive, and well-behaved plants suited to the site and with attractive forms and textures through all seasons.

More critical to the therapeutic garden are concerns about possible toxic exposures for especially vulnerable users. Poisonous plants, whether cultivated ornamentals or weedy interlopers, should not be accessible to users in or near the garden. Examples include rhubarb (leaves), delphinium, yews, foxglove, deadly nightshade, golden chain tree (seeds), and daphne; for more, see Turner and von Aderkas (2009) or visit Cornell University's excellent website, ansci.cornell.edu/plants. Also to be avoided are plants with prickly leaves, thorns, or barbs. Many grasses appear soft, but their blade edges inflict slivery cuts. Screening plants for potential allergens is more difficult, as allergic responses vary from user to user and determining specific sensitivities is usually not practicable; but a planting plan can avoid including those species that commonly cause the most troublesome allergic responses. The worst culprit in the Northwest is the aspen, a tree that disperses large amounts of allergy-producing pollen. Mold, another allergen common in most gardens, is a specific concern to those with suppressed immune systems. Mold can be minimized or killed by designing the garden for good air circulation and direct exposure to sunlight. Mold is found in compost, where it actually helps to break down wood and leaf fibers. If a composting bin or pile is used, site it away from gathering spaces. Those with mold allergies should not participate in the making or spreading of compost in the garden.

Topsoils and composted amendments should be certified as free of toxins, in particular heavy metals such as lead, arsenic, or mercury. Organic composts, mulches, and fertilizers are recommended to build the tilth of soils and deliver nutrients effectively and gradually. Toxic pesticides are unhealthy for people and for wildlife and have no place in a therapeutic garden. Safer controls are available for most insects and diseases. Good culture—appropriate plants, nourishing soils, and a thriving population of beneficial insects—is the best way to maintain a healthy garden.

Cultivating a garden offers participants many physiological, social, and emotional benefits. For individuals in senior care facilities or in rehabilitation clinics and for those with degenerative illnesses, the physical activity of deadheading, digging, raking, mulching, or weeding can tune fine and gross motor skills and improve balance, coordination, strength, and stamina, resulting in increased energy and better sleep habits. The sensory experience—aromas and textures—can rekindle fond memories. As participants exchange their expertise and ask questions, they teach and learn from each other, improving the quality of their engagement. For older adults or those marginalized due to their conditions or disabilities, intellectual satisfaction has positive health consequences. The social interactions that spontaneously occur while cultivating the therapeutic garden can effortlessly pull participants out of isolation. A sense of accomplishment and heightened self-esteem can unfold as participants see the value of their contribution to the garden. Not many activities are as hopeful and forward-looking as gardening.

But not all maintenance tasks are appropriate for volunteers. The participant's capacity and the challenge of the task need to be well matched. Experienced guidance will train gardeners to find challenging exercise in the work without overstressing muscles and joints. Some conditions—those which impair balance, reduce mobility, or limit strength or reach; attention or sensory deficits, such as blindness or loss of sensation in hands and feet; processing issues or impulsivity—may preclude some volunteers from participating in the full range of maintenance tasks. Still others may be photosensitive and will need to have cover, or work in a shade garden.

Hardscape Maintenance

Hardscape maintenance is important in all gardens, not only in therapeutic settings. It involves ground surfaces, surface textures, stability, seating, drainage, water features, irrigation, and lighting.

GROUND SURFACES

Maintenance of ground surfaces is critical for those with mobility, balance, and wayfinding issues. Of chief concern is any settling or heaving of the ground plane that results in uneven terrain: the garden will not be a destination if users perceive an uncertain passage, such as a risk of falling or of twisting an ankle. At one hospice facility the drylaid entry landing into the garden had subsided only half an inch, but the patients could not get their drip line supports over the grade change so they stopped using the garden. The problem starts with poor compaction of the base materials (gravel or sand) or existing substrate soils; the paving material then subsides, creating a trip hazard. Though it can sometimes be traced to a fault during the installation phase, the problem can occur even with proper installation after intensive storms, when water can undermine the paving. After the contractor is gone, the maintenance or facilities personnel will have to rectify it. For concrete or stone pavers, the fix is relatively easy. It will be necessary to remove the paving in the problem area, replace the gravel or sand, and recompact the soil subbase, then reinstall the base courses and paving. If the uplift of the pavers is caused by frost heave, remove the paving and excavate deeper into the native soils, lowering the subbase until it is below the frost line. Frost depths can be found on most county or local municipality websites. Add and compact more base material, the gravel or sand, and reset the paving. The problem is more complicated when settling or heaving occurs underneath a concrete slab. The heaved concrete must be removed by saw-cutting, and then the substrate problem can be fixed as just described. A new patch of concrete can be poured, matching the wearing course in color and texture.

SURFACE TEXTURES

Particular attention is needed to preserve traction on surfaces to avoid injury and overcome lack of confidence in navigating the garden space. For example, people with mobility problems or declining or impaired vision, such as those recovering from a stroke or those with glaucoma, will need a reliable, firm footing. Design protocol dictates avoiding ultra-smooth finishes on stone or concrete pavers or terrazzo. Brick, which can quickly grow moss in shady, moist conditions, is not a good choice in rainy climates or on the north side of a building. Regular maintenance treatments to remove and repel the formation of moss and algae, also found on wood decking, may be needed. With age, pavers can wear and lose the textures that prevent slipping and will need to be replaced.

Warning strips done with tape products will peel over time and need to be replaced. Warning strips of differing textures, patterns, or materials can achieve the same result: those with poor eyesight, or who are unable to read color changes, will be alerted by footfall that a change in grade or texture is about to occur.

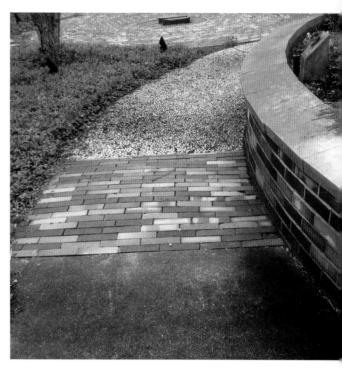

For change of surface textures to be a safe and reliable rehabilitation element in the garden, careful maintenance procedures need to be followed to keep the transitions smooth, the joint spaces filled, and the surfaces level and free of debris.

STABILITY

Railings, seats, and tables will need regular checks for stability. Users with impaired balance, sensation, or coordination will bear down hard on railings, seats, and armrests, needing them for support and stability. A railing or armrest that bounces or rocks even slightly will be interpreted as unreliable and unsafe, discouraging its use. Connection points, joints, and mechanical fasteners will need testing and tightening. Rusting, peeling paint, or other roughening of the railing may be uncomfortable for users as the result of certain medications or illnesses, or for those with highly sensitive and delicate skin such as the elderly, small children, people with sensory processing disorders, or those undergoing chemotherapy. Rust should be removed and the metal evaluated for structural integrity. The area can either be refinished with a primer and paint, or removed and replaced with a new component. Decks, sheds, and overhead structures such as arbors and pergolas should be inspected for failed decking or framing members, with similar attention to fasteners and finishes.

SEATING

Seating should be installed for positive drainage, with no water pooling on the seat surface. Benches and chairs with wood slats need regular inspection, particularly in the fall when leaf debris can dam the voids between the slats, inhibiting drainage and causing moss to grow. Oil, stain, and paint should be reapplied as needed to ensure that the wood is protected and preserved.

DRAINAGE

Drains need to be checked and cleared of leaf litter, soil, or silts. Any puddles that form will be difficult for users to navigate, and, in cold regions, they can freeze and cause a slip hazard. Drain gates must be secured to ensure they stay level with the surrounding paving. Any subsidence of paving around drains needs to be corrected immediately, so those using wheeled mobility devices, walkers, crutches, and canes can move smoothly and safely and users of all abilities can enjoy the garden.

WATER FEATURES

A water feature is often the central element in a therapeutic garden. Clients and users rank them as highly valuable during participatory design input and focus groups sessions, and indeed their benefits are many.

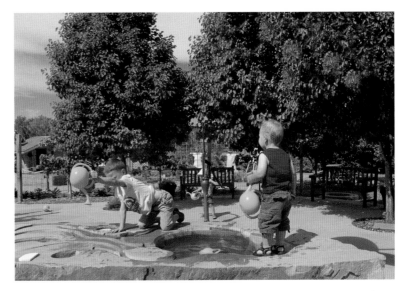

Water is irresistible to most children. Keeping water play safe is not only a concern for supervising adults (especially those who are watching toddlers) but an important maintenance priority.

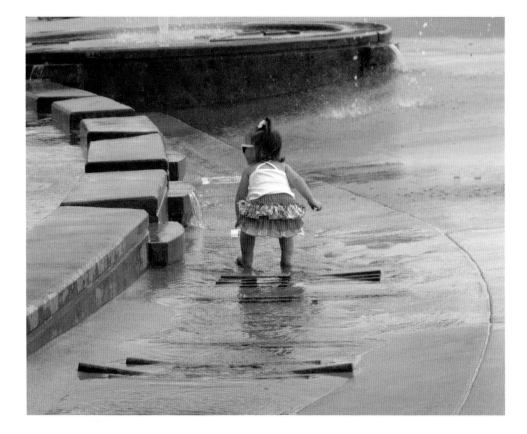

Water enriches the senses of touch, sight, and hearing in primary and evocative ways. Occupational therapists use water for hydro- and play therapy with adults and children. Many water features are artfully ornamented with mosaic tiles or equally colorful concrete or stucco surfaces; they become landmarks in the garden and gathering points for people to meet, socialize, and escape from the stresses of medical or cold and institutional environments.

While dynamic, desirable, and engaging, water features are not without significant maintenance challenges. Contact with water is a concern for people with compromised immune systems, so the water quality must meet the local health standards. When water (including its spray) is contaminated and carries unsafe levels of bacteria, the consequences can be serious, even deadly; several cases of Legionnaire's disease, for example, have been linked to the water supply at hospitals, long-term care facilities, and rehabilitation centers.

Fountain professionals who understand all technical aspects of filtration systems should be consulted for safe and sound fountain design. The

Playing in water, touching it, and frolicking in it is fun and therapeutic. Careful maintenance ensures that the experience will also be safe.

facility and maintenance personnel will be responsible for maintenance following the manufacturer's recommendations, and these procedures—periodic replacement of the filtration materials (sand, charcoal, gravel), cleaning the pipes, disinfection of the pool surfaces, including waterfalls, channels, and spillways—validate the warranty period. If chlorine is used, it should be tested daily and adjusted to meet local health department standards. If any signs of algae, dirt, or odors appear, the fountain should be shut down, the areas in question cleaned, and the system checked for blockages. Some facilities have moved away from chlorinated, closed water reuse models and instead are dumping the water or using it for irrigation. While this ensures a safer water feature, it is a costly and unsustainable use of water. If UV systems are used in lieu of chemical treatments, the fixture must be periodically checked and the water tested for bacteria or other contaminants.

The most troubling aspect of water features for owners and designers has been the potential failure of the waterproofing systems, but the

Whether naturalized or highly stylized, water features require regular, stringent, and ongoing maintenance to run smoothly and safely.

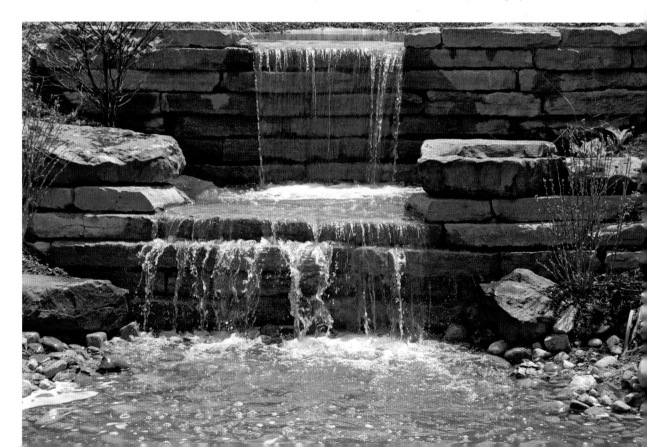

technology is being updated, and new materials are entering the market all the time. Most liners have improved flexibility and can maintain a good seal under the stress of slight variations caused by expansion of the concrete or ceramic base materials. Still to be understood is how well they will perform over time with exposure to UV, abrasion, and temperature changes. Owners should periodically test water features for minor leaks, which can often be solved with minimal intervention before major repair is required; this can be done by filling the feature and checking for small air bubbles, or marking the line of water and observing if over time the level decreases.

IRRIGATION

In many parts of the country, the irrigation system is drained and winterized so pipes do not break when temperatures dip below freezing. In the spring when it is brought back online, the system is checked for leaks, loose connections, and clogs. In pop-up systems, where watering heads are visible above ground, leaks are easier to locate than in subsurface or surface drip systems. In subsurface systems, with emitter pipes four to eight inches below grade, leaks are often evident only when the plants wither from lack of water or when there is puddling around the failed pipe; once located by excavation, the damaged section of pipe is removed and replaced. In surface drip systems, the "micro" emitter heads are so small the orifice often gets clogged; the head will need to be detached to remove the blockage. Again, plant stress is an indicator, but the heads and pipe connections should be inspected yearly.

LIGHTING

The trend in exterior lighting is toward LED lights, which last much longer than fluorescent or incandescent but still need periodic bulb replacement. Most spot- or fountain lights have protective glass lenses that tend to get coated or clouded; these will need to be cleaned seasonally to ensure intensity of light. Many spotlights are flexible and can be adjusted to throw their light up or down; the locking screw commonly loosens over time and needs readjusting to eliminate glare or to redirect the beam, as originally intended. Some light timers will need to be adjusted for seasonal changes; use light sensors to eliminate this maintenance task.

The Costs

The costs of maintenance are primarily the costs of labor and material replacement and repair. They can be assessed as a balance between the short-term costs of construction and the long-term costs of maintenance. Two cases illustrate the complexity of such decisions. An arbor, for example, may be warranted to provide shade and support for a bench swing and flowering vines, not to mention the therapeutic and symbolic benefit of passing through it, as a metaphor of moving from an illness or loss into recovery. In most conditions an arbor made of untreated wood will last five to 10 years, depending on the tree species. If built with second-growth cedar, depending on the grade and if using paints or stains, the arbor will last 10 to 15 years; most of these toxic treatments, however, have associated health issues and might be inappropriate for users with compromised immune systems or who are sensitive to smell. To avoid or reduce outgassing of toxic chemicals, consider using one of the many green low-VOC paint and stain products on the market. As an alternative, the arbor might be made of powder-coated steel. Powder-coating is essentially pigment melted and fused onto the metal; a powder-coated arbor offers a greater period of service, 20 to 30 years, but it will be considerably more expensive to fabricate.

Weighing a low-maintenance strategy, such as replacing a grass lawn with a meadow, presents similar complexities. In time a meadow may offer a cost savings, but initially it may require greater labor (planting and weeding) and material costs (all those perennial plugs) than the grass alternative. Without maintenance considerations in the initial budget, most clients will want to have as much built, at as little cost, as possible. Thinking down the road to the long-term condition of the garden is critical so that the garden will not degrade and become a liability for users or become unusable. It is important to recommend that the client allocate a part of the budget for an endowment to fund long-term maintenance.

AFTERWORD

We end where we began, by recounting the merits of being in nature and the importance of good design to maximize connections with nature—that is, being outside, doing what one wants and needs to do, in a safe and enriching environment that improves physical, emotional, cognitive, and spiritual health and well-being. Meditating in a walled garden or immersing oneself in a contemplative forest walk are ancient means of curing the mind and body, and we now have a body of evidence-based research from varying disciplines to verify that such practices have positive therapeutic outcomes.

Undeniably, our lives are increasingly frenetic, overstimulating, and for many, depersonalizing. The rigors of daily life are constant: imagine the compounding and unbalancing effects of stress on those facing trauma, marginalization, and debilitating illness. Being in nature, in a garden that heals, can counteract the overwhelming challenges people face every day. Looking for and finding balance and meaning in life is critically important. The salutary benefits that a therapeutic garden may provide can be a way back to coherence from seemingly incoherent situations.

As special places, these gardens do not belong only to those who "are sick"—nor should they have an exclusive partnership with healthcare venues. Unquestionably therapeutic gardens in hospitals are valuable, and for those facing disease and illness, the therapeutic garden can and must be a place of solace. But extending their benefits beyond traditional healthcare institutions means those benefits will reach often-overlooked populations who need them just as much.

Gardens appear in many forms, serving many needs: they provide us with food, beauty, and refuge; we learn, play, and exercise in them. For those displaced by poverty or fleeing violent environments where threats are pervasive, the garden becomes a valuable connection to home. It is a safe place to learn about the growing customs of a new place or to memorialize and include familiar plants, cultural shrines, and other positive elements from a grounding past. A therapeutic garden can counter the effects of food deserts and malnourishment. It can be a welcoming place to feel a part of something bigger than oneself, to come together to grow not just food but the body, the mind, the spirit. It can be a place to learn new skills and start over again. For the shattered, the garden can become a place of rebirth, and for the abandoned, a place of hope and renewal. The garden itself can be a desirable and motivating place to heal from physical and emotional wounds and illness. In therapeutic gardens people can receive rehabilitation and participate in counseling sessions. Gardens transform degraded environments and at-risk communities into healthier, more productive social and ecological systems. Neighbors that gather in the garden can then go out and on to strengthen community ties. No matter the form, venue, or intended purpose, a therapeutic garden has the capacity to gracefully envelope and support those who use them. They are places to experience restoration, rejuvenation, and gratitude.

A collaborative design approach fosters gardens with optimal salutary benefits. Approaching therapeutic garden design from an interdisciplinary perspective allows designers to find a well-balanced mix between the socio-cultural and biophysical aspects of any project. It is an important way to ensure that the human-centered connection between people and nature, the doing and performance aspects of the garden, are the primary focus of the project. It is also a way to ensure that the garden is designed with the utmost compassion and respect for those who use it. A common ground to meet the challenges of people-centered design is to follow universal design principles, which are, at heart, about equity for all who use the therapeutic garden, wherever or for whomever it may be installed.

Landscape architects have the power to create places that can elicit powerful transformations. These designed spaces play an important role in restoring well-being, repairing the damaged earth, and increasing the health of our youth and elderly, through the production of nutritious food and by providing opportunities for play. That those less fortunate may benefit from your designs, those traumatized or downtrodden may find safe and welcoming places to rest and rebuild their spirits, is an exciting prospect. It is our hope that your therapeutic gardens will be places of inspiration, where people can come together for support and connection, or where they can find the physical and emotional space to be alone and experience a safe and nurturing environment, a place that alleviates, even briefly, the stresses and uncertainty of a situation.

The four principles discussed at the beginning of this book offer a framework to establish design goals—and to evaluate a project once completed. Do the participants have a greater sense of control? Does the design elicit positive feelings of escape, of "being away"? Does it provide people with opportunities to regain control of their emotions and to refocus their attention? Does the design foster a sense of belonging and connection, qualities of familiarity that create deeper connections to place and improve self-confidence? Through heightened interactions with nature and sensorial nourishment, the user's emotional state can be improved and stress and anxiety reduced. Finally, has your design supported increased opportunities for movement and physical exercise for all?

Great design is responsive design. Responsive design must be compassionate design. Acknowledging one's limitations is critical to creating responsive proposals. Understanding what we do not know enables us to seek new knowledge. A participatory design process offers insights into the needs, limitations, aspirations, and hopes of the intended users. This process will offer a deeper understanding of cultural beliefs and rituals, the nuances and effects of an illness, and the dietary, recreational, and spiritual needs of a specific community. In the end, you design places to attract and nurture all comers—people, plants, animals, and insects. If it does not foster a healthy life for all the intended beneficiaries, no matter how well it photographs, the design has not succeeded. Sometimes design requires a deep meditation and focused singular attention. But in the larger scheme of things, most of landscape architecture needs to be a shared endeavor that includes other disciplines, community members, clients, and stakeholders. This shared mind experience ensures that the design exceeds clients' needs. Through therapeutic garden design, we have an opportunity to serve a higher cause, a cause that represents the values that are at the core of a vibrant and healthy society. Uphold these values and approach each therapeutic garden design challenge with passion and confidence as you create the changes necessary for a healthy and sustainable future.

References

Adams, William H. 1991. *Nature Perfected*. New York: Abbeville Press.

Alzheimer's Disease International. 2010. *World Alzheimer Report*. alz.co.uk/research/files/WorldAlzheimerReport2010.pdf.

American Horticultural Therapy Association. 1995. *Therapeutic Garden Characteristics*. ahta.org/sites/default/files/attached_documents/TherapeuticGardenChracteristic_0.pdf.

American Occupational Therapy Association. 2013. *About Occupational Therapy*. aota.org/en/About-Occupational-Therapy.aspx.

American Psychiatric Association. 2013. *Diagnostic and Statistical Manual of Mental Disorders DSM-V-TR*. 5th ed. (text revision). Washington, D.C.: American Psychiatric Publishing.

Antonovsky, Aaron. 1987. *Unraveling the Mystery of Health*. San Francisco: Jossey Bass.

———. 1996. The salutogenic model as a theory to guide health promotion. *Health Promotion International* 11(1): 1.

Ayres, A. Jean. 2005. *Sensory Integration and the Child*. 25th anniv. ed. Los Angeles: Western Psychological Services.

Babbs, Helen. 2011, February 22. *Soil Stained Survivors*. theecologist.org/green_green_living/gardening/781586/soil_stained_survivors_how_gardening_is_helping_those_caught_up_in_the_balkan_wars.html.

Baio, Jon. 2014. Prevalence of autism spectrum disorders among children aged 8 years. *Surveillance Summaries* 63(SS03): 1–21. cdc.gov/mmwr/preview/mmwrhtml/ss6302a1.htm?s_cid=ss6302a1_w.

Barnard, Victoria L., et al. 2009. *Trauma and Physical Health*. London: Routledge.

Bean, Robert. 2004. *Lighting*. Oxford: Architectural Press.

Berger, Ronen, and Mooli Lahad. 2010. A safe place. *Early Child Development & Care* 180(7): 889–900.

Bodin, Maria, and Terry Hartig. 2003. Does the outdoor environment matter for psychological restoration gained through running? *Psychology of Sport and Exercise* 4:141–153.

Calkins, Meg. 2013. *The Sustainable Sites Handbook*. Hoboken, N.J.: John Wiley & Sons.

Castriota, Louis J., Jr. 2013. *Leg Up! The Courage to Dream*. New York / Tulsa: Blooming Twig.

Center for Universal Design. 2008. *The Principles of Universal Design*. ncsu.edu/ncsu/design/cud/.

Centers for Disease Control and Prevention. 2012. *Overweight and Obesity*. cdc.gov/obesity/data/adult.html.

Chawla, Louise. 2003. Bonding with the natural world. *NAMTA Journal* 28(1): 133–154.

Cimprich, Bernadine, and David L. Ronis. 2003. An environmental intervention to restore attention in women with newly diagnosed breast cancer. *Cancer Nursing* 26:284–292.

Coon, Jo, et al. 2011. Does participating in physical activity in outdoor natural environments have a greater effect on physical and mental well-being than physical activity indoors? *Environmental Science & Technology* 45(5): 1761–1772.

Coppedge, Clay. 2012, August 31. *Keyhole Gardening Offers Alternative*. countryworldnews.com/news/headlines/1183-keyhole-gardening-offers-alternative.html.

Cornelissen, Frans W., et al. 1995. Object perception by visually impaired people at different light levels. *Vision Research* 35(1): 161–168.

De Young, Raymond. 2013. Environmental psychology overview. In Ann Hergett Huffman and Stephanie R. Klein, eds., *Green Organizations*. New York: Routledge.

Diette, Gregory, et al. 2003. Distraction therapy with nature sights and sounds reduces pain during flexible bronchoscopy. *Chest* 23(3): 941–948.

Donahue, Emily. 2010, August 10. *Seeds for Peace*. saratogian.com/articles/2010/08/22/news/doc4c71e15ee1e3f235677280.txt.

Dyment, Janet E., and Anne C. Bell. 2008. Our garden is colour blind, inclusive and warm. *International Journal of Inclusive Education* 12(2): 169–183.

Gill, Jessica, et al. 2009. PTSD. *The Nurse Practitioner* 34(7): 30–37.

Gómez, Juan-Carlos, and Beatriz Martín-Andrade. 2005. Fantasy play in apes. In Anthony D. Pellegrini and Peter K. Smith, eds., *The Nature of Play*. New York: Guilford Press.

Gonzalez, Marianne, et al. 2010. Therapeutic horticulture in clinical depression. *Journal of Advanced Nursing* 66(9): 2002–2013.

Graham, Heather, et al. 2005. Use of school gardens in academic instruction. *Journal of Nutrition Education & Behavior* 37(3): 147–151.

Gruson, L. 1982, October 19. *Color Has a Powerful Effect on Behavior, Researchers Assert*. nytimes.com/1982/10/19/science/color-has-a-powerful-effect-on-behavior-researchers-assert.html?pagewanted=all.

Helphand, Kenneth. 2006. *Defiant Gardens*. San Antonio, Tex.: Trinity University Press.

Herzog, Thomas R., and Glenn E. Kutzli. 2002. Preference and perceived danger in field/forest settings. *Environment & Behavior* 34(6): 819–835.

Herzog, Thomas R., et al. 2003. Assessing the restorative components of environments. *Journal of Environmental Psychology* 23:159–170.

Holmgren, David. 2002. *Permaculture*. Victoria, Australia: Holmgren Design Services.

Hopper, Leonard, ed. 2007. *Landscape Architectural Graphic Standards*. Hoboken, N.J.: John Wiley & Sons.

Ikiugu, Moses N. 2004. Instrumentalism in occupational therapy. *The International Journal of Psychosocial Rehabilitation* 8:109–117.

Irvine, Katherine N., and Sara L. Warber. 2002. Greening healthcare. *Alternative Therapies in Health and Medicine* 8:76–83.

Jaffe, Aaron. 2011, October 31. *Youth Program Plants Seeds for Success*. http://seattletimes.com/html/localnews/2016658868_gardenworks01m.html.

Jiler, James. 2006. *Doing Time in the Garden*. Oakland, Calif.: New Village Press.

Julian, Warren Gordon. 1983. The design of the visual environment of the aged partially sighted. *Architectural Science Review* 26(3/4): 112–115.

Kahn, Peter H., and Stephen R. Kellert, eds. 2002. *Children and Nature*. Cambridge, Mass.: MIT Press.

Kaplan, Rachel, et al. 1998. *With People in Mind*. Washington, D.C.: Island Press.

Kaplan, Rachel, and Stephen Kaplan. 1989. *The Experience of Nature*. New York: Cambridge University Press.

——. 2005. Preference, restoration, and meaningful action in the context of nearby nature. In Peggy F. Barlett, ed., *Urban Place*. Cambridge, Mass.: MIT Press.

Kaplan, Stephen. 1995. The restorative benefits of nature. *Journal of Environmental Psychology* 15:169–182.

——. 2001. Meditation, restoration, and the management of mental fatigue. *Environment & Behavior* 33:480–506.

Kielhofner, Gary. 2009. *Conceptual Foundations of Occupational Therapy Practice*. 4th ed. Philadelphia: F. A. Davis Company.

Kirkwood, Niall. 1999. *The Art of Landscape Detail*. Hoboken, N.J.: John Wiley & Sons.

Kuo, Frances E., and William C. Sullivan. 2001a. Environment and crime in the inner city. *Environment & Behavior* 33(3): 343–367.

——. 2001b. Aggression and violence in the inner city. *Environment & Behavior* 33(4): 543–571.

Kuo, Frances E., and Andrea Faber Taylor. 2004. A potential natural treatment for attention-deficit/hyperactivity disorder. *American Journal of Public Health* 94(9): 1580–1586.

Kuyk, Thomas Jeffrey, et al. 1998a. Visual correlates of obstacle avoidance in adults with low vision. *Optometry and Vision Science* 75(3): 174–182.

——. 1998b. Visual correlates of mobility in real world settings in older adults with low vision. *Optometry and Vision Sciences* 75(7): 538–547.

Li, Fuzhong, et al. 2005. Improving physical function and blood pressure in older adults through cobblestone mat walking. *Journal of the American Geriatrics Society* 53:1305–1312.

Linden, Sonja, and Jenny Grut. 2002. *The Healing Fields*. London: Frances Lincoln.

Louv, Richard. 2005. *Last Child in the Woods*. Chapel Hill, N.C.: Algonquin Books.

Luck, Rachael. 2003. Dialogue in participatory design. *Design Studies* 24(3): 523–535.

Malhotra, Savita, and Partha P. Das. 2007. Understanding childhood depression. *The Indian Journal of Medical Research* 125(2): 115–129.

McGeary, Don, et al. 2011. The evaluation and treatment of comorbid pain and PTSD in a military setting. *Journal of Clinical Psychology in Medical Settings* 18(2): 155–163.

Minelli, Alessandro. 1996. *The Botanical Garden of Padova (1545–1995)*. Venice: Marsilio Publishers.

Mitchell, Richard, and Frank Popham. 2008. Effect of exposure to natural environment on health inequalities. *The Lancet* 372(9650): 1655–1660.

Mollison, Bill. 1988. *Permaculture*. Tasmania, Australia: Tagari Publications.

Mollison, Bill, and David Holmgren. 1981. *Permaculture One*. Davis, Calif.: International Tree Crop Institute USA.

Nakamura, Ryuji, and Eijiro Fujii. 1990. Studies of the characteristics of the electroencephalogram when observing potted plants. *Technical Bulletin of the Faculty of Horticulture of Chiba University* 43:177–183. (In Japanese with English summary.)

Newman, Oscar. 1996. *Creating Defensible Space*. huduser.org/publications/pdf/def.pdf.

Norman, Sonya B., et al. 2006. Associations between psychological trauma and physical illness in primary care. *Journal of Traumatic Stress* 19(4): 461–470.

Olds, Clifton C. 2008. *The Japanese Garden*. learn.bowdoin.edu/japanesegardens.

Ottosson, Johan, and Patrik Grahn. 2005. A comparison of leisure time spent in a garden with leisure time spent indoors: on measures of restoration in residents in geriatric care. *Landscape Research* 30:23–55.

Park, Bum Jin, et al. 2010. The physiological effects of shinrin-yoku (taking in the forest atmosphere or forest bathing). *Environmental Health and Preventive Medicine* 15:18–26.

Picker Institute and Center for Health Design. 1999. *Assessing the Built Environment from the Patient and Family Perspective*. Walnut Creek, Calif.: The Center for Health Design.

Pitch, M., and C. Bridge. 2006. Lighting your way into home modifications. In *Selected Papers from the 2006 International Conference on Aging, Disability and Independence, Florida* 181–191.

Pretty, Jules, et al. 2005. The mental and physical health outcomes of green exercise. *International Journal of Environmental Health and Restoration* 15(5): 319–337.

Rainey, Reuben M. 2010. The garden in the machine. *Site/Lines* 5(2): 14–17.

Rodale, Robert. 1987. *Organic Gardening*. Westminster, Md.: Ballantine Books.

Schweitzer, Marc, et al. 2004. Healing spaces. *Journal of Alternative and Complementary Medicine* 10:71–83.

Sharp HealthCare. 2013. *Therapeutic Gardens Provide Peaceful Pathways to Recovery for Mental Health Patients.* sharp.com/mesa-vista/therapeutic-gardens.cfm.

Sheldon, Cohen, et al. 2012. Chronic stress, glucocorticoid receptor resistance, inflammation, and disease risk. *PNAS* 109(16): 5995–5999.

Sklarew, Bruce H., and Harold P. Blum. 2006. Trauma and depression. *The International Journal of Psychoanalysis* 87(3): 859–861.

Soong, Grace, and Jan E. Lovie-Kitchin. 2001. Does mobility performance of visually impaired adults improve immediately after orientation and mobility training? *Optometry and Vision Sciences* 78(9): 657–666.

Sternberg, Esther M. 2009. *Healing Spaces.* Cambridge, Mass.: Harvard University Press.

Stigsdotter, Ulrika A., and Patrik Grahn. 2002. What makes a garden a healing garden? *Journal of Therapeutic Horticulture* 13:60–69.

Taylor, Andrea F., et al. 2002. Views of inner nature and self-discipline. *Journal of Environmental Psychology* 22(1–2): 49–63.

Tidball, Keith G., and Marianne E. Krasny, eds. 2014. *Greening in the Red Zone.* New York: Springer.

Tuke, D. Hack, and Geo. H. Savage, eds. 1881. Reviews: advantage of the farm as a source of occupation. *Journal of Mental Science* 576. (ebook ed.)

Turner, Lori W., et al. 2002. Influence of yard work and weight training on bone mineral density among older U.S. women. *Journal of Women and Aging* 14(3/4): 139–148.

Turner, Nancy, and Patrick von Aderkas. 2009. *The North American Guide to Common Poisonous Plants and Mushrooms.* Portland, Ore.: Timber Press.

Ulrich, Roger S. 1984. View through a window may influence recovery from surgery. *Science* 224:420–421.

——. 1991. Effects of health facility interior design on wellness. *Journal of Health Care Design* 3:97–109.

Ulrich, Roger, et al. 1991. Stress recovery during exposure to natural and urban environments. *Journal of Environmental Psychology* 11(3): 201–230.

van den Berg, Agnes E., and Mariette H. G. Custers. 2011. Gardening promotes neuroendocrine and affective restoration from stress. *Journal of Health Psychology* 16(1): 3–11.

Wagenfeld, Amy. 2012. Health through HOrTiculture™. *Home and Community Health Special Interest Section Quarterly* 19(2): 1–4.

Wagenfeld, Amy, and Bernice Buresh. 2012. Ergonomic gardening. *OT Practice* 17(9): 8–11.

Wagenfeld, Amy, Connie Roy-Fisher, and Carolyn Mitchell. 2013. Collaborative design: outdoor environments for veterans with PTSD. *Facilities* 31(9/10): 391–406.

Walch, Jeffrey, et al. 2005. The effect of sunlight on postoperative analgesic medication use. *Psychosomatic Medicine* 67:156–163.

Walker, Haley. 2009, 20 November. *Inmates Harvest Food, Savings, Education and Jobs from Jail Gardens.* greatlakesecho.org/2009/11/20/inmates-harvest-food-savings-education-and-jobs-from-jail-gardens/.

Weinstein, Netta, et al. 2009. Can nature make us more caring? *Personality and Social Psychology Bulletin* 35:1315–1329.

Wells, Nancy, and Gary Evans. 2003. Nearby nature. *Environment & Behavior* 35:311–330.

Westmacott, Richard. 1992. *African-American Gardens and Yards in the Rural South.* Knoxville: University of Tennessee Press.

Whall, Ann L., et al. 1997. The effect of natural environments upon agitation and aggression in late stage dementia patients. *American Journal of Alzheimer's Disease* 12(5): 216–220.

Wilson, Edward O. 1984. *Biophilia.* Cambridge, Mass.: Harvard University Press.

Winterbottom, Daniel. 1998. Casitas. *Urban Agriculture Notes.* Vancouver: City Farmer (Canada's Office of Urban Agriculture).

——. 2007. Casitas. *Journal of Mediterranean Ecology* 8:77–86.

——. 2008. Garbage to garden. *Children, Youth and Environments* 18(1): 435–455.

——. 2014. Developing a safe, nurturing and therapeutic environment for the families of the garbage pickers in Guatemala and for disabled children in Bosnia and Herzegovina. In Keith Tidball and Marianne E. Krasny, eds., *Greening in the Red Zone.* New York: Springer.

Acknowledgments

FROM DANIEL: I owe much to Miriam Talasnick, my mother, who, while lying in her hospital bed with the chemo slowly dripping into her vein, directed my attention to the window and commented on how noble and comforting the enormous white pine dominating the view was. I didn't know then how prophetic her statement would become until I devoted my career to creating environments that might sustain others who had unfortunately to share my fear, resolution, and grief. To my wife, Carol, who has so often stood beside and guided me, I am profoundly grateful. To my daughter, Nina, who always shines so bright, and to those from whom I have learned so much: Clare Cooper-Marcus, Teresia Hazen, Kenny Helphand, Hanley Denning, Sally Schauman, Vesna Šendula Jengić, and Luka Jelusic. To Jeremy Watson, who taught me courage and humility while coping with the devastation of war; to all the other students, who have nourished and joined me on this journey; and to Pat Logerwell, who introduced me both to veterans in need and those wonderful wise women at Nikkei Manor.

FROM AMY: I would like to thank my husband, Jeffrey Hsi, for his enduring patience, support, and love. To our son, David, deepest gratitude for the unending joy and light you bring to my life. I love you dearly. To my parents, Morton Wagenfeld and Jeanne Wagenfeld, thank you for raising a daughter who contrary to your aversion to the garden, fell headfirst into it. Who would have thought? To my siblings, Eric, David, and Ellen, playing gardener at your homes is the best. To my talented photographer niece Ajna Wagenfeld, I offer huge thanks for your patience, encouragement, and instruction. To my beloved late graduate school advisor Carol Harding, you gave me the greatest gift of all: the courage and conviction to believe in myself and reach for the stars. I miss you every day. To all my occupational therapy colleagues who have enthusiastically followed the writing process and cheered me on as I forge new paths and connections, a big giant thank you.

Our combined and heartfelt thanks to David Kamp, principal of Dirtworks, PC. We are profoundly honored to include your eloquent foreword and images in our book. You work magic with your words and your designs.

To the talented and dedicated staff at Timber Press—Andrew Beckman, Juree Sondker, Franni Farrell, and Sarah Milhollin. Together, we made an idea come to fruition. It has been an outstanding experience to work with you all.

Finally, we wish to acknowledge and thank the many other people and organizations who generously and variously contributed to the book: African Elder Farming Program at Rainier Beach Urban Farm & Wetlands (Michael Neguse), Arvada Community Garden (Bill Orchard), Barry Rustin Photography, Beacon Food Forest (Melody Wainscott), Beacon Hill Nursery School (Lucinda Ross), BHA Design (Angie Milewski), Boston Children's Hospital (Andrea Duggan), Bronson Methodist Hospital (Susan Watts), Brenda Parent, Cadence Design (Gage Couch and Rebecca Bradley), Canuck House, Carter School (Marianne Kopaczynski), Cilla Kitay, Dana-Farber Cancer Institute (Robbin Ray), David Berarducci Landscape Architecture, Dirtworks, PC (Deanna Medina), Dirt Works Incubator Farm (Nikki Seibert), Dowling Community Garden (Peter Schmidt), Elisabeth Refn, Esther Greenhouse, Farmacy Garden (Renee Reichart), FNN of Goodwill Columbus, Ohio (Margaret Tabit), Franklin Park Conservatory and Botanical Gardens Growing to Green Program (Bill Dawson), Freedom from Torture (Katy Pownall), Gabriela Fojt, Gardens on Spring Creek (Christine Ginnity), Gray Mockingbird Community Garden (Brian Kirsch), Growing a Greener World (Joe Lamp'l), Grow Dat Youth Farm (Johanna Gilligan), Hafs Epstein Landscape Architecture (Mark Epstein), HGA Architects (Nissa Tupper), Hali'imaile Community Garden (Lori Feroldi), Hmong Village Community Garden (Ghia Xiong), Holly D. Ben-Joseph, Hope in Bloom (Roberta Hershon), Inver Hills–Metropolitan State Interdisciplinary Community Garden and Orchard (August Hoffman and Barbara Curchack), Jane McCabe, Jeavons Landscape Architects (Mary Jeavons), Johansson Design Collaborative (Sonja Johansson), Kang Lee, Karen Jacobs, Kevin LaChapelle, Leg Up Farm (Louie Castriota), Massachusetts General Hospital (Ryan Chapman), Mauricio Rubio, Mahan Rykiel Associates (Lydia Stone), MC Haering, Michela Tolli, Mikyoung Kim Design, National AIDS Memorial Grove (John Cunningham and Steve Sagaser), Nikkei Manor (Lisa Waisath), Palm Beach County Schools (Erica Whitfield, Ted Gliptis, and Melissa Rothmel), Quatrefoil, Inc. (Brian Bainnson), Ruth McLean, Safe Passage (Dave Holman), Salk Institute (Rhiannon Bruni), Scripps Health (Lisa Ohmstede), Seattle Tilth (Liza Burke), Seattle Youth Garden Works (Ron Servine), SEN, Inc. (Yoshisuke Miyake), Stephanie Murphy, St. Louis Children's Hospital (Abby Wuellner), Studio Sprout (Connie Roy-Fisher), Susan Sorensen, The Horticultural Society of New York (Hilda Krus), The Lord's Place (Diana Stanley), Therapeutic Landscapes Network (Naomi Sachs), Thrive (Alyson Chorley), Tri-City Medical Center (Becky Orozco), University of Oklahoma (Thomas Woodfin), Urban GreenWorks (James Jiler), VA Puget Sound Fisher House (Pat Norikane Logerwell), Veterans Farm (Adam Burke), Westley Design (Michael Westley), Yachats Community Garden (Marje Takei).

Photography and Image Credits

Index

About the Authors

Daniel Winterbottom, RLA, FASLA, is professor of landscape architecture at the University of Washington and earned his MLA from the Harvard Graduate School of Design. Daniel's research is in landscape as a cultural expression, ecological urban design, and restorative/healing landscapes in the built environment. His firm, Winterbottom Design Inc., focuses on designing healing/restorative gardens.

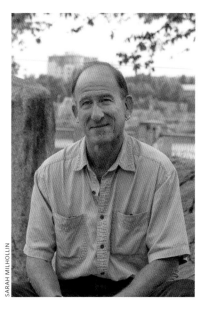

SARAH MILHOLLIN

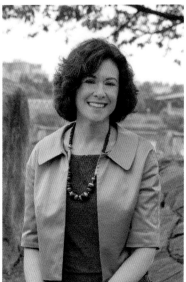

SARAH MILHOLLIN

Amy Wagenfeld, PhD, OTR/L, SCEM, CAPS, an occupational therapist, educator, researcher, and master gardener, brings a unique perspective to her work by blending occupational therapy, horticulture, and design to make gardens and gardening possible for a wide range of adults and children. She is on the faculty in the department of occupational therapy at Rush University and has a landscape design consultation practice.